CONTENTS

PREFACE

What do I think of the NHS Plan?

That's the question I'm most often asked these days. A better question is what do you think about it? You've got the tough job. You've got to deliver it. Oh, yes. No hiding place! There isn't any part of the NHS that won't be poked and polished, in some way, by the time the Plan is fully implemented!

That's the issue, isn't it? No part of the NHS untouched!

To be honest, when the plan was published, on the first read I was disappointed. In retrospect, I think I was wrong to be disappointed. I was looking for something different. For me 'reform' means throwing the whole lot up in the air and starting again. Slash and burn! Typical Lilley!

The NHS Plan is not about that. This is a different approach. The NHS Plan is built upon the type of good stuff that is going on all over the place, every day in the NHS – right now. The type of good stuff that NHS managers, medics, nurses and others are kind enough to show me as I make my way around our health services. I've seen a lot of what is in the NHS Plan already – some of it years ago! Best practice, joint working, measured outcomes . . . The sort of great stuff that comes from people working together, sharing ideas and having a single aim.

So, I was disappointed. No smell of burning, nothing demolished! Then I started to think about the Plan differently. If every hospital in every nook and cranny of the NHS was working as well as the best, in everything they do, we'd have a service that would do us proud. This is just that opportunity.

Usually, when the NHS comes up with something new, it ends up with more pilots than British Airways. In this Plan there is very little to pilot – someone is flying this idea, this best practice, this different approach, somewhere, already. Nothing experimental. These ideas deserve to be used, everywhere. Taken together they are a recipe for reform.

It's a long-range plan, with a sub-text. When someone challenges the performance of the NHS, it will give the politicians the opportunity to say 'We've put more money on the table, consulted the staff and devised the plan. Give it time, it's up to them'. The trick will be not to lose sight of the key objectives and to make sure they are delivered – all of them.

Is the Plan top-down management? Sure. Lots of targets, new frameworks, protocols, national standards. Of course it's top-down. And, in a national administration why shouldn't

W225

A TOOL KIT FOR THE
NHS PLAN

Roy Lilley

RADCLIFFE MEDICAL PRESS

30·00

© 2001 Roy Lilley

Radcliffe Medical Press
18 Marcham Road, Abingdon, Oxon OX14 1AA

British Library Cataloguing in Publication Data

A catalogue record for this book is available from the British Library.

ISBN 1 85775 484 0

Typeset by Joshua Associates Ltd, Oxford
Printed and bound by Hobbs the Printers, Totton, Hants

head office tell you what they want done. The trick is giving folk enough freedom to deliver. That's the challenge for ministers.

The next brouhaha will be over implementation. There is no implementation plan and there won't be until the Modernisation Agency (a new outfit) gets to grips with it. Remember somebody is already doing most of it. So you have the opportunity to find out who they are and ask them how they did it! If it's really new ground, have a go! You can't be wrong!

There are things you may not like. Things that may challenge what you do and what you believe. If the NHS is to survive it has to be more customer friendly, less self-obsessed and more open to evaluation. This will hurt parts of the medical establishment and bring three cheers from other places. This is an opportunity.

And this is all we've got for the next 10 years! A pile of money and a heap of good practice. Before you jump off the top, remember that the mind is like a parachute. It works better when it's open. Happy landings!

Roy Lilley
August 2000

ABOUT THE AUTHOR

Roy Lilley is a former NHS Trust chairman. He now writes and broadcasts on NHS and social care issues.

This is the eighth book in his best selling tool kit series and the latest addition to the list of books he has written on management, the health service and social matters.

Roy Lilley is a favourite speaker on these topics and divides his time between speaking engagements in the UK, Europe and the US, writing books and articles for newspapers and magazines, riding his bicycle and disappearing off on his boat.

He can usually be found at www.roylilley.co.uk

This book is, in part, an apology to the umpteen people who have seen me speak on NHS issues, reforms and the NHS Plan, and have asked me for a copy of my slides. If I've forgotten to send them – here they are. It's all in here somewhere!

It's also dedicated to the army of NHS workers, who once again will be challenged to deliver a new agenda. The fact that they so seldom fail is the biggest compliment to their skills and talents that I so much admire.

For ATR, in the hope that I continue to feature in her national plan!

ABOUT THIS BOOK

This is not a textbook, not a how-to-do-it book, nor an academic book. It's an indispensable book for people who need to get a fast handle on what the NHS Plan is all about and the issues it raises.

It's for people who might, rightly, be asking the question – how is all this going to affect me? And, it's for people who will be helping to lead the process that will result in a big shake-up of health and health services.

It consists of chunks from the original plan, commentary, some things to think about, challenges, ideas and thoughts on implementation. It includes opinion, assumptions, unfair guestimates, commonsense and gossip.

It also has:

 THINK BOXES which raise issues about the Plan and allied matters.

 HAZARD WARNINGS – things to look out for.

 Stuff to make a **NOTE** of, think about in more detail and work through – either on your own or with your colleagues.

 . . . and the ubiquitous coffee break and rest!

So, this is a book that the Secretary of State would probably burn. A book that is not supposed to be taken seriously, a book to write on, rip pages out and dip in and out of.

A book aimed at demystifying government aims, targets, ambitions and gobbledegook. A book I hope you'll find fun, useful and worth the modest investment you have made to my *Get on the Beach Fund*.

Happy days!

SECTION 1

What happened, who did what and why?

The NHS used to be awash with committees, these days we have teams. Got a problem? Have a team.

The Prime Minister dropped his bombshell on 22 March 2000. Unprecedented for a Prime Minister, Tony Blair made a personal statement to the House of Commons about the state and the future of the NHS. Wearing his underpants over his trousers, Super Tony said he was going to sort out the NHS – in a single stride!

Seriously, this was important stuff. PMs don't usually make statements like that – that's what they've got Secretaries of State for. However, the modernisation of the NHS is high on the New Labour list of things to do. New money in the NHS must mean new ways of doing things. This is what Tony Blair told Brian Groom, the political editor of the *Financial Times*:

It's pointless putting more money into public services unless it's accompanied by reform.

Mr Blair pledged 'a different vision for the health service'.

FT 16 March 2000

Different vision? Reform? What does this mean? Well, the Prime Minister set out five challenges for the NHS.

They became known as the '5 Ps':

- **Partnership** – making all parts of the health and social care system work better together and ensuring the right emphasis at each level of care

- **Performance** – improving both clinical performance and health service productivity

- **Professions** – increasing flexibility in training and working practices and removing demarcations, in the context of major expansion of the healthcare workforce

- **Patient care** – which has two components: ensuring fast and convenient access to services and the system; and empowering and informing patients so that they can be more involved in their own care

- **Prevention** – tackling inequalities and focusing the health system on its contribution to tackling the causes of avoidable ill health.

So, what was the up-shot? You've guessed it. Six teams!

The action teams were focused on how NHS modernisation could be taken forward.

The key members of the modernisation action teams are:

Prevention and Inequalities

- Professor Liam Donaldson, Chief Medical Officer (Chair)
- Rabbi Julia Neuberger, Chief Executive, King's Fund
- Jim Johnson, Chairman, Joint Consultants' Committee
- Professor Sir Michael Marmot, Professor of Epidemiology and Public Health, University College London
- Dr Nick Hicks, Strategy Unit, Department of Health

Partnership in the Health and Social Care System

- John Hutton MP, Minister of State, Department of Health (Chair)
- Christine Hancock, General Secretary, Royal College of Nursing
- Dr Ian Bogle, Chairman of Council, British Medical Association; General Practitioner, Liverpool

- Jo Williams, President, Association of Directors of Social Services; Director of Social Services, Cheshire
- Gavin Larner, Strategy Unit, Department of Health

Patient Care (Speed of Access)

- Lord Hunt, Parliamentary Under Secretary of State (Lords), Department of Health (Chair)
- Barry Jackson, President, Royal College of Surgeons; Consultant Surgeon, St Thomas' Hospital
- Tony Newton OBE, Baron Newton of Braintree; Chair, North East Essex Mental Health NHS Trust
- Professor Chris Ham, Strategy Unit, Department of Health

Patient Care (Empowerment)

- Gisela Stuart MP, Parliamentary Under Secretary of State for Health, Department of Health (Chair)
- Sarah Mullally, Chief Nursing Officer
- Melinda Letts, Chairman, Long Term Medical Conditions Alliance; member of the Commission for Health Improvement
- Karlene Davis, General Secretary, Royal College of Midwives
- Jo Lenaghan, Strategy Unit, Department of Health

Performance and Productivity

- Yvette Cooper MP, Parliamentary Under Secretary of State for Public Health, Department of Health (Chair)
- Stephen Thornton, Chief Executive, NHS Confederation
- Professor Mike Pringle, Chairman of Council, Royal College of General Practitioners; Professor of General Practice, University of Nottingham
- Professor Don Berwick, President and Chief Executive, Institute of Healthcare Improvement; Clinical Professor of Paediatrics and Head of Healthcare Policy, Harvard Medical School
- Professor Liam Donaldson, Chief Medical Officer
- Richard Murray, Strategy Unit, Department of Health

Professions (Workforce)

- John Denham MP, Minister of State for Health, Department of Health (Chair)
- Professor Sir George Alberti, President, Royal College of Physicians; Professor of Medicine, University of Newcastle upon Tyne

- Bob Abberley, Head of Health, UNISON
- Professor Jill Macleod-Clark, Professor of Nursing and Deputy Dean, Faculty of Medicine and Health, University of Southampton
- Nick Ross, Broadcaster
- Professor John van Reenen, Strategy Unit, Department of Health.

Further members, including frontline clinicians and managers who have been at the forefront of modernisation in their local hospital or health community, will be added over time.

So that's alright then . . .

 ## Make a Note

Do you think this list is just the usual suspects? Government always looks to the establishment for a view. What else can they do? Do the great and good speak for you? Did your professional organisation contact you and ask for your views? Taken against the background of the other consultation tools used in this exercise, is this about as comprehensive as it gets?

If you were going to organise the committees, who would you have asked to take part?

Consultation – tell us what you think

Consultation, consultation, consultation – that's the name of the game. But it has all been done before.

The most famous consultation process, involving the public and asking them how health services should be organised, took place in the state of Oregon in the US.

The Oregon Health Services Commission (OHSC) asked the public to prioritise services that would be included in the US Medicaid system. Through surveys and facilitated workshops, OHSC used community values to establish a priority-setting process. At the time it was regarded as very sexy stuff and just about every health management guru went to have a look at what was going on. Even the ones who didn't go had an opinion!

With the benefit of 20/20 vision that comes with the wisdom of hindsight, the Oregon experiment has been largely discredited. Discredited? Yes. Too harsh a word, perhaps? Downgraded might be better. It has been denounced. The majority of consultees were middle class Americans who were not affected by Medicaid and had their own private medical insurance provision.

In 1992, New Zealand had a go at consultation. This is much closer to the exercise used by the UK government. The National Health Committee in New Zealand was set up to advise the government on the priorities for funding health and disability services. So they:

- produced a booklet and distributed it through libraries and schools
- and held public meetings,

with the aim of finding out which services the public valued the most. Six areas were identified:

1 mental health services
2 services for children
3 integrated community services (with special attention to the needs of the Maori population)
4 ambulance services
5 hospice services
6 rehabilitation services.

In other words, everything! So, the government decided to go with children's services, mental health services and integrated community care.

The New Zealand Committee followed up with another booklet asking which services should be publicly funded. Through a series of small groups and stakeholder workshops they got together with the elderly, ethnic groups, teenagers, people on low incomes and disabled people.

Out of this work emerged a priority-setting framework. The work is on-going and includes the regular circulation of 10 000 newsletters, inviting opinions. Ten thousand may not seem much but bear in mind that New Zealand, in population terms, is only about the size of a UK NHS region.

The New Zealand approach, in guru-speak, is called a multi-method approach and is similar to the approach used in the UK. It's a good approach if you want to take in a wide range of views but only has currency if the participants can see their input influencing policy. If they don't, everyone soon gets fed up and goes home!

Margaret Hosburgh a member of the New Zealand Committee said:

> It's our responsibility to make decisions having considered as much information from as many different sources as possible in the time available. Before any consultation exercise, it should be made clear that the contributions that are forthcoming will not, of themselves, be binding. But it's equally important to show the steps that were taken and the information that was given weight in reaching the final decision. If the workings of a sensible decision can be set out clearly, the decision has a greater chance of being accepted, particularly by those who made some contribution to it.

Source: Hosburgh M (October 1996) *The Public's Values and Public Choices*. Stockholm Conference on Priorities in Healthcare.

Seems to me that our NHS has a way to go.

Here's the problem.

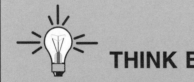

THINK BOX

Consultation is a waste of time. Either the government has a policy for the NHS – in which case why waste all this time and money on a useless consultation exercise – or it doesn't.

If it doesn't they are incompetent. We elected them to sort out the NHS (remember the slogan 'Vote Labour, you've got 24 hrs to save the NHS'?). What's the policy, what are you going to do? Don't ask us, you're the government.

Which do you think is right?

Three wishes

As part of the government's modernisation agenda it embarked upon a potentially massive consultation programme to seek the views of the public. The government wanted to know what the public thought was important about the NHS and asked them for three things they thought needed changing.

Twelve million forms were printed and distributed at NHS offices, surgeries, hospitals, supermarkets and other retail outlets. The aim was to find out how the extra £20bn earmarked for the NHS over the next four years would, in the view of the public and NHS staff, best be spent.

The exercise cost £500 000 and the response was disappointing. Only 200 960 replies were received. I make that about £2.40 each.

The replies were analysed by *Broadata* based on a structure drawn from past ideas and suggestions expressed by staff and public. However, this has translated the replies into a range of headings many of which are meaningless, such as 'Doing things differently'.

Many have dismissed the exercise as a sham and an expensive one at that! Was it a waste of money? If you take the view that the more you find out about what your staff and customers are thinking the better it is, then you might be persuaded that the money was well spent.

The interesting fact is not that the NHS staff want more pay and the public isn't too fussed about the idea, and that the NHS wants people to take more care of their health and the public doesn't seem to think too highly of that idea – the big issue is the difference between public and NHS perception on the same topics. Under some headings the NHS seems a million miles away from its customer.

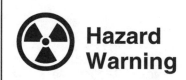

Hazard Warning

The survey boffins will tell you that this was a small sample of self-selecting middle class, middle aged people and is therefore unrepresentative and next to use-less! Others might say that these are the views of folk who are really interested in the topic and that we should listen to them – *'yer pays yer money and yer takes yer chances!'*

 Time for a coffee and a look at the data . . .

Who bothered to reply?

Twelve million questionnaires distributed – here's who responded.

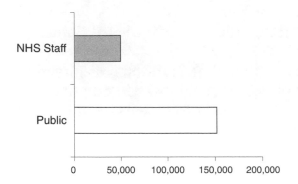

NHS:

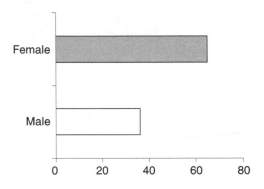

The public:

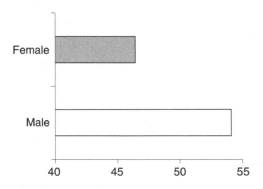

. . . and over 74% of the public were over 45 years old.

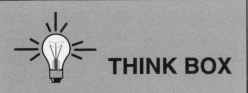

THINK BOX

Is the poor response rate significant? When you consider the fact that the NHS is hardly ever out of the headlines, why did so few people take the opportunity to reply?

Is the poor response from staff significant? Are they fed up, can't be bothered, don't think it'll make any difference and see no way out of the mess!

The higher level of male responses may be significant. Generally, it's women who most frequently 'interface' with the NHS, and conventional wisdom holds that men neglect their health and present with symptoms later.

Why then is there a higher response from the men?

Too middle aged to be meaningful? Bear in mind that it's the kids and the seniors who make most use of healthcare services.

NHS staff

What did the people at the coalface have to say?

Are these killer issues?

		Agree	Disagree
28%	**Capacity:** • more doctors and nurses • more pay for other staff • more staff • more nurses		
22%	**Quality:** • improve training • improve management skills • improve mental health services		
10.5%	**Local services/access:** • improve linked healthcare • improve community care • improve/modernise primary care		
9.9%	**Doing things differently:** • reduce administration • improve funding structure • reduce management		
8.3%	**Prevention/education:** • more information for public • earlier diagnosis • educate public about their responsibilities		

		Agree	Disagree
8.3%	**Treatment of staff:** • support NHS staff • aim at better staff retention • reduce junior doctors' hours		
7.4%	**Waiting:** • reduce it generally • reduce wait to see specialist • more flexible appointment times		
1.9%	**Patient-centred care:** • more holistic care • care more for elderly • NHS staff explain more		
1.8%	**National variation in service:** • provide more performance information • end variations in access to drugs • improve staff accountability		
0.9%	**Politics:** • take politics out of the NHS • more staff consultation • be more honest about waiting lists		
0.33%	**Charges:** • abolish prescription charges • free dental charges		

The public

OK, what did the customers say?

Are these killer issues?

		Agree	Disagree
27%	**Capacity:** • more nurses • more pay for staff • more doctors		
20%	**Waiting:** • reduce wait to see GP or consultant • reduce waiting generally • provide flexible appointments		
16%	**Doing things differently:** • bring back matron(!) • reduce admin and bureaucracy • improve funding structure		
8%	**Patient-centred care:** • improve communication skills • care more for elderly • more holistic care		
7%	**Quality of NHS staff and care:** • improve GPs' diagnostic skills • provide regular training for nurses • improve cancer services		

		Agree	Disagree
6%	**Consumer experience:** • improve cleanliness • end mixed sex wards • improve food		
4%	**Local services/access:** • more cottage hospitals • improved community care • provide better transport		
3%	**Treatment of NHS staff:** • reduce junior doctors' hours • reduce nurses' hours • support NHS staff		
3%	**National variations:** • equal access for all • end variation in access to drugs • provide more performance information		
3%	**Prevention/education:** • invest money in prevention • more info on public education • educate the public about its responsibilities		
2%	**Politics:** • be more honest about waiting lists • take politics out of NHS • be honest about mistakes		

		Agree	Disagree
2%	Charges: • reduce prescription charges • abolish prescription charges • charge foreign patients		

What else did they do?

Although the survey got all the headlines, the Gods of Whitehall were busy with other stuff too. They had a four-pronged attack on consultation.

Workshops

Leeds and London were the venues for two one-day workshops. Around 100 people were recruited as a 'typical mix' of the local population. There was small and large group discussion and the participants were invited to vote on key issues and draw up recommendations for the modernisation action teams.

Patient and User Organisations

Telephone interviews with 30 of the main NHS user and patient groups, plus a series of seminars.

Open Access

This is guru-speak for the 12 million leaflets inviting NHS staff and the public to give their three 'top tips' for making the NHS ace-tastin', superfizzin' and all lovely. There was also a website.

Focus Groups

Ah, the focus group – always a favourite amongst the white wine drinkers of Islington! There were 10 groups, involving 80 people, held across England. Each group included a particular category of people.

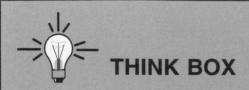

THINK BOX

Did you have your say? Do you know anyone who did? If you didn't, here's your chance. What three things would you have told the Secretary of State to do in order to sort out the bit of the NHS where you work?

1

2

3

Now take your reply, fold it up and throw it away – because you're too late. Or pin it on the board in your office to make out that you're still interested!

Let's see it their way. . .

Where do NHS staff and the public agree, or disagree?

More staff and more pay:

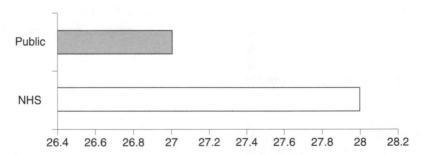

Reduce waiting:

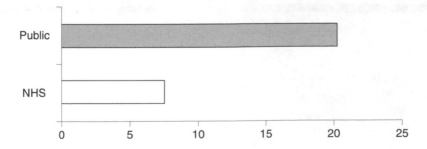

Improve quality:

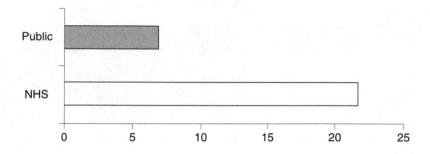

More patient-centred care:

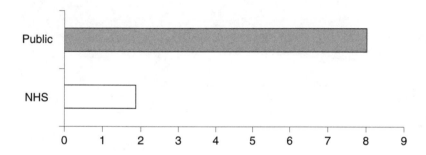

Reduce national variations in care (postcode issues):

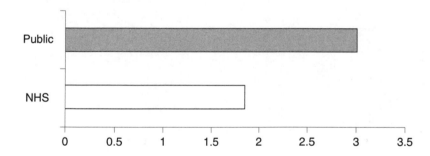

Prevention and education:

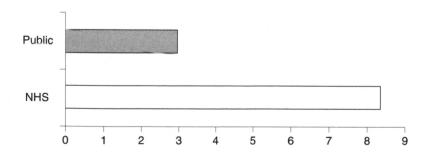

Reduce/abolish charges (prescription and dental etc.):

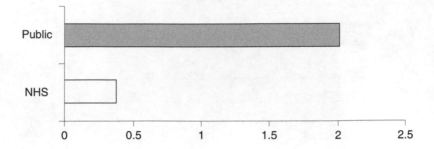

More local services/improve access:

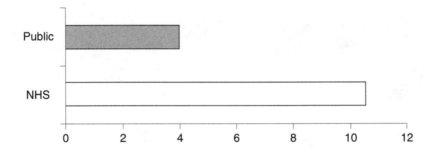

Improve treatment of NHS staff:

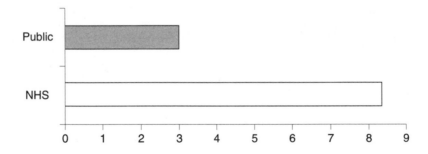

Do things differently and reduce admin etc.:

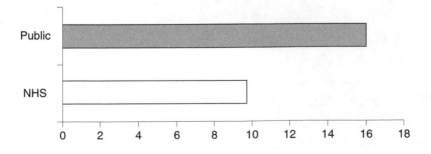

What can we make of all this?

Take a good look at the variations between NHS staff aspirations and opinions, and those of the public. Is it fair to conclude that patients want the NHS to do things differently and the NHS is reluctant to embrace change? The NHS wants the public – overweight, on the couch and smoking a fag – to take greater care of their own health. Thank you! The public is worried about 'post code rationing' – the NHS hardly considers it. The NHS wants more wages and staff – the public (who pays for it through taxes) is not so keen!

Imagine the NHS as a business, say, NHS Plc. The modern business is fanatical about customer value, recognising customer need and fulfilling customer expectation. Lord King, the former head of British Airways, once said: 'It used to be enough to think that the customer was king. That is no longer enough. The modern business must recognise that the customer is God!'

Business used to say that it was necessary to move closer to their customers – now they talk of being 'entwined' with their customer. Business used to say 'what can we sell and how much can we get for it?' Today, the message is 'what do customers want and how much will they pay for it?'

So, once again think of the NHS as a business. From the results of this survey, does the NHS look like a 'business' that is fanatical about customer value, is it 'entwined' with its customers? Or does it look like the NHS is going off in one direction and the public in another?

The NHS wants to provide local services, the public seem less fussed about it. The public is concerned about patient-centred care, the NHS hardly seems to know what it means!

OK, so the NHS is not a business but it does have customers. The public pays for the NHS through taxes and that makes them a customer. Millions of men and women go to work, slave all day and find nearly a third of their pay packet has been pick-pocketed by the taxman. They also pay goodness knows how much more tax through so-called stealth taxes (indirect taxation). Whatever your view about taxation, the redistribution of wealth and funding public services, the unavoidable fact is that public services should reflect public needs and expectations – because the public pays for them.

Is it fair to conclude from the consultation exercise that the NHS doesn't have a clue what its customers want and lives in a world of its own?

Make a Note

Consider the results of the public consultation exercise. Look at the divergence of importance attached to key elements, between the NHS and the public.

Are the differences important? Should the NHS go all out to meet public expectations or are they unrealistic, striking at the fundamentals of the NHS and, in the long run, not good for the NHS? Or should strategies be put in place to work to a greater convergence of view?

Consider your view and develop strategies that would work on a local level to deliver the necessary changes.

The NHS is a special place. It's the world's biggest nationalised industry – everything that BT once was, British Airways used to be and the Post Office does not want to be. For some strange reason, NHS employees have a schizophrenic mindset. Think about it this way:

- they complain like hell if they see a waiter's finger print on a wine glass, but are blind to their complicity in the causes of fatal, hospital-acquired infections by not washing their hands

- they kick up a stink if a new pair of socks has a manufacturing flaw, but close ranks on holes in treatments and dangerous practice from colleagues and work mates

- if their holiday charter flight is late they open their wallets for compensation, but shut their eyes to cancelled admissions, appointments and over-run clinics

- NHS staff expect to shop at midnight and buy mortgages on-line, but they fight shy of working in weekend clinics and moan endlessly about NHS Direct, which enjoys a 98% public approval rating!

Why don't NHS staff bring their expectations to work?

 Make a Note

Do you agree that NHS staff are prepared to let things go in the NHS, that they would never put up with in the world outside?

If you do, make a list of the possible reasons for it. Does it start with disempowerment, do staff feel unable to change things, does it centre on a 'nothing to do with me, nothing I can do about it' attitude?

What is stopping real customer focus in the NHS? Do you have trouble with the word 'customer'? Are you more comfortable with 'patient'?

Here's a list of some of the factors that mark out a successful business – do they have any place in the NHS? How does the NHS stack up against these hallmark standards?

Hallmark standard	NHS	Business
On top of the problem, a focused sense of urgency and a feeling of having a grip on what's going on.	Too big and cumbersome for staff to really feel empowered.	Management lines are short. In one of the world's biggest corporations, Microsoft, all staff can e-mail Bill Gates, the Chairman, direct and are only five management layers away from him – worldwide.
A proper regard for the role of the 'customer' and their needs, and a recognition that without customers the organisation would not exist.	No incentive to think of patients as customers as there is no competition. The public has to sit around for hours in A&E, or wait for operations – they have no option.	Urgent requirement to capture customers – competition is too fierce to be sloppy.
External pressures and targets.	NHS head office is the government which has a re-election agenda in which the NHS is at the centre. Circulars and guidance are generally prescriptive and de-motivating.	Head office sets targets for the organisation as a whole. There is a feeling that everyone is working for each other, towards a common objective.
Leaders with a clear sense of vision.	Most NHS staff cannot name the chief executive of the NHS, and in a recent survey the majority of NHS Trust staff could not name the chairman or pick out the chief executive from a collection of photographs.	Leaders are visible, known and share their vision and objectives. Richard Branson at Virgin pays some of the lowest salaries in the industry but his staff are loyal and talented. Branson makes everyone feel part of the team and makes a point of getting out and about in the organisation.
A feeling of 'I'm involved' and 'I can make a difference'.	Few NHS staff ever feel they can make a difference. Organisations employ thousands of people and staff 'get lost' in the system. Few Trusts have meaningful staff suggestion schemes. Innovation can invite failure and that can be career limiting in a blame culture environment.	Staff are routinely encouraged to make suggestions on efficiency and improvements, and are rewarded.

Hallmark standard	NHS	Business
Rewards to encourage good performance with particular regard to customer service.	NHS pay is confused. Professions have different review bodies, and collective bargaining reinforces differentials. Good performance is seldom rewarded.	It's rare to find a private sector company that does not have an incentive or reward programme. They are invariably based on turnover or sales targets which reflect customer volume and satisfaction.
A determination to cut out red tape and bureaucracy that gets in the way of service.	The NHS moves towards a centralist management model, and control and bureaucracy breed red tape. Poor use of information technology to manage information in the system.	Successful organisations are flat structures and make a point of streamlining procedures, particularly in the use of information technology.
A commitment to swift change to reflect moving circumstances – revolution not evolution.	Pilot sites and trials are used – the hallmarks of an organisation which is conservative and unwilling or unprepared for change.	Businesses re-brand frequently, re-design products and move swiftly to reflect changing customer expectations and values.

Developed from the work of Jenny Rogers, Management Futures Consulting.

 Make a Note

Agree or disagree? What's it like where you work? Take the hallmark points and apply them to where you work.

Did we need to do all this?

On the day of the announcement of the NHS Plan, Sky TV asked its viewers to phone vote on the question:

'Will the NHS Plan cure the ills of the NHS?'

Here's what the viewers said . . .

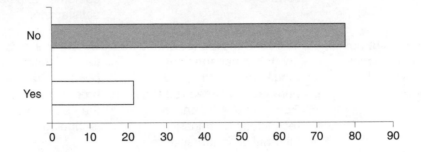

So, not much confidence there then!

I guess we knew all that. However, in June 2000 the Department of Health published some of its own data, which included this little nugget!

The percentage of the public saying that the '[health] system works pretty well, only minor changes are needed':

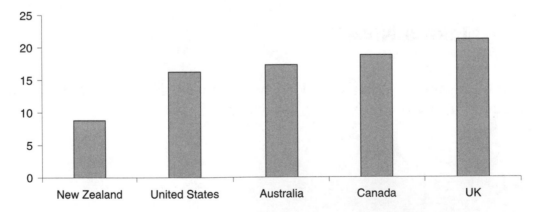

Source: Commonwealth Fund 2000

Mmmm, I'll leave you with a coffee whilst you figure all this out!

Well, after all that we ended up with:

Trallaaaaaaa . . .

The NHS Plan

A plan for investment
A plan for reform

Presented to Parliament by the
Secretary of State for Health
By Command of Her Majesty

July 2000

> Except that it wasn't. Presented to Parliament by the Secretary of State for Health, I mean.
>
> It was presented to Parliament by the Prime Minister.
>
> What is the significance of this? Just Tony wanting to be associated with 'eye-catching ideas', or a real political heavyweight push towards delivery?

In fairness, the Prime Minister did pay tribute to his Right Honourable Friend, the member for Darlington, Alan Milburn, for all the hard work he and his colleagues had put into the plan, but I wonder how it feels to sit in the House of Commons and see your moment in history pinched from under your nose?

Is this Tony's plan or is it Alan's plan? Is it even the NHS's plan? Is it our plan? Is it your plan? Do you feel a sense of ownership in the plan? Do you feel part of delivering it? Do you feel responsible for it?

> Clement Atlee, the PM of the day, didn't try and steal the show when Aneurin Bevan introduced his plans for the NHS – he stood back and let Bevan unveil them to the House of Commons.

Isn't one of the key elements of motivating the delivery of change the idea of making everyone feel part of it? The government understands all that. Look at who they got to sign up to the document . . .

Prof Sir George Alberti *President*
Royal College of Physicians of London

Barry Jackson *President*
Royal College of Surgeons of England

Prof Mike Pringle *Chairman of Council*
Royal College of General Practitioners

Dr Ian Bogle *Chairman of Council*
British Medical Association

Stephen Thornton *Chief Executive*
NHS Confederation

Dr Michael Dixon *Chairman*
NHS Alliance

Christine Hancock *General Secretary*
Royal College of Nursing

Bob Abberley *Head of Health*
UNISON

Karlene Davis *General Secretary*
Royal College of Midwives

Dr Jenny Simpson *Chief Executive*
British Association of Medical Managers

Sir Jeremy Beecham *Chair*
Local Government Association

Harry Cayton *Chief Executive*
Alzheimer's Society

Dr Peter Smith *Chair*
National Association of Primary Care

Rabbi Julia Neuberger *Chief Executive*
King's Fund

Prof James McEwen *President*
Faculty of Public Health Medicine

Natalie Beswetherick *Chair*
Allied Health Professions Forum

Melinda Letts *Chairwoman*
Long Term Medical Conditions Alliance

Barbara Meredith *Policy and Communications Manager* Age Concern London and The Patients' Forum

Delyth Morgan *Chief Executive*
Breakthrough Breast Cancer

Diana Whitworth *Chief Executive*
Carers' National Association

Eoin Redahan *Director of Public Relations* The Stroke Association

Bob Gann *Director*
The Help for Health Trust

Paul Richard Streets *Chief Executive*
Diabetes UK

Sir Alexander Macara *Chairman*
National Heart Forum

Sir Nicholas Young *Chief Executive*
Macmillan Cancer Relief

Now, here's the question – why did they sign up to the document? Were they flattered to be asked? Was it an ego thing? All of those nice trips to London and a walk up Downing Street to tell the kids about?

Or was it a sincerely held belief that this plan could change the NHS? It's a question worth asking because, as this book was being written, the BMA had already started to distance itself from the plan. Peter Hawker, Chairman of the BMA Consultants' Committee, told the *Guardian*:

> The plan showed a 'profound lack of understanding of the work they [consultants] do'. And their [the government's] only new idea was 'an ill-conceived and vindictive attack on new consultant's freedom to work outside the NHS'.

Guardian 28 July 2000

. . . well, we can see where his first loyalty lies! Not a great start!

Liam Fox, the shadow health secretary, told the same newspaper:

> This was a wonderful opportunity for Tony Blair to move from political to clinical priorities. Unforgivably he has put his own political survival before the survival of patients.

Well, he would say that. So, who's right?

Christine Hancock, CEO of the Royal College of Nurses, said:

> [the plan] was a 'survival plan that puts patients first and tackles the hardest issues facing the health service'.

Guardian 28 July 2000

This quote is in stark contrast to the 'bitter disappointment' voiced by Gordon Lishman, Director General of Age Concern, about the government's rejection of the Royal Commission recommendation that the NHS should pay for personal care in residential homes. It's easy to argue, Christine, that here's a 'hard issue' not tackled and patients' needs not put first.

Hey wait a minute! Go back one page! No, don't bother, here's the important bit

. . . from the signatories list:

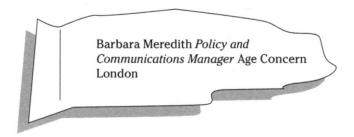

> Barbara Meredith *Policy and Communications Manager* Age Concern London

Do you think Lishman and Meredith talk to each other? They are both from the same organisation. One has signed up to the reform package and one sees it as a 'bitter disappointment'. What do you think? The great and the good can't seem to agree!

Make a Note

Think about the issue of ownership. Organisations representing you have probably signed up to the plan. So, it's yours whether you like it or not! How will you address the issues of ownership where you work? Without doubt there will be things in the plan that will impact on you and how you work. If you are responsible for a team, devise ways of instilling a sense of ownership in these changes. How will you make everyone feel part of what is going on?

The BMA can't seem to sell the idea. Here's an extract from a joint statement from the RCGP and the BMA:

> The guarantee of access, within 48 hours of request to GPs, by 2004, could only be achieved by a much greater investment in the capacity of general practice than presently proposed.

So what's wrong boys? Can't you read? Didn't you look at what you were signing up for? You look like a double glazing salesman's dream!

Head BMA honcho Ian Bogle attacked the proposals to move doctors remuneration to another format as:

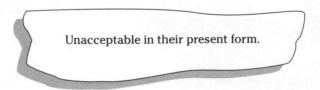

> Unacceptable in their present form.

Ian, you're a lovely chap but do you need new glasses?
Spec-Savers are doing a deal right now . . .

It didn't get any better. Here's the lead story from the *Daily Telegraph* on the 3 August:

FAMILY doctors dealt a major blow to the government's plans for the National Health Service yesterday, criticising them as disappointing and unworkable.

In the first concerted attack on the plan announced by Tony Blair last week, they warned that the pledge of an extra 2000 GPs over four years could not meet current or future patient demand. They said they would resist any move to change their traditional contract.

An alliance of the Royal College of General Practitioners and the GPs' Committee of the British Medical Association said the government had got its sums wrong on GP numbers and that they would resist any moves to 'victimise' doctors in a sole practice.

Under the plan, by 2004 GPs will be expected to see a patient within 48 hours of a request for an appointment. All patients should be able to see a nurse the next day. However, the doctors said there were limits to the degree to which nurses could relieve their workload.

The family doctor service forms a central part of Labour's plans to modernise the health service, with the creation of groups of GPs in Primary Care Groups and the development of more powerful Primary Care Trusts. The NHS Plan contained a surprise for the GP body: a clear government intention to change the traditional GP contract in favour of a new payment scheme currently being piloted.

In the next two years, about a third of GPs would be expected to have accepted the new Personal Medical Services (PMS) contract, the plan said. This opens the door to a salaried GP service in place of their traditional status as independent practitioners and is expected to be strongly resisted.

In the statement from the Royal College and the BMA, GPs accepted that some features of the old contract needed reforming but said there was no evidence that PMS schemes offered better or most cost-effective care.

They also expressed 'profound disappointment at the limited planned expansion of the general practice workforce' which would not cope with current demand let alone new targets imposed. The BMA said there needed to be a 30 per cent expansion of GP numbers.

The GPs also questioned the government's expansion figures. The plan's promise of an extra 2000 GPs in England is a seven per cent increase on the current 28 500. The GPs said this represented an increase of 1.6 per cent a year.

Dr Hamish Meldrum, joint deputy chairman of the BMA GPs' Committee, said: 'Before the plan was announced we were already getting an extra 0.9 per cent so the real increase is only 0.7 per cent a year. We are now seeing over 70 per cent of training places going to women, who will want time off for their families. We estimate that for every GP who retires we will need to enrol 1.5 or 1.6 GPs to replace them.'

The plan called for appraisal of all GPs, which would mean taking time away from patients. Prof Mike Pringle, chairman of the RCGP, said: 'We need more GPs just to cope with current patient demand. But the NHS Plan proposes an appraisal system by 2001. This will need one whole-time doctor for every 50 GPs – an extra 600 doctors a year.'

Both bodies said they were wary of the proposal to expand the PMS contracts and would resist any move to impose them. Dr Meldrum said: 'We do not believe it's in the patients' or the profession's interests for there to be an unseemly rush into PMS. There should not be any coercion either implicit or explicit to do so. All GPs choosing the PMS option must do so voluntarily.

'The government expectations are totally unworkable and unrealistic. Many GPs are angry. There is a lot of disillusion and resignation about – both metaphorical and literal.'

. . . and yes, you're right, the BMA is a signatory to the document! Look . . .

Dr Ian Bogle *Chairman of Council BMA*

SECTION 2

Let's get started

Because you've been wise enough to get hold of a copy of this book you won't have to sit down and plough through the 145 pages of text in the original document. You can instead leave it to me (*and the Editor – Ed!*) to pick out the important bits. You do, of course, run the risk that what I think is important may not be important to you. In which case, you better read the plan and this book!

Anyway, here are a couple of important bits from the introduction:

> . . . the government has decided to make an historic commitment to increase the funding of the NHS over the next four years. The Prime Minister's announcement in March of large, sustained investment in the NHS provides the funding that doctors, nurses, dentists, therapists, managers and other staff have called for over the years.

> More money is, however, only the starting point. The challenge is to use the resources available to achieve real benefits for patients and to ensure that the NHS is modernised to meet modern public expectations. That is why in announcing the increase in funding for the NHS, the Prime Minister set five challenges that needed to be addressed: partnership; performance; professions and the wider NHS workforce; patient care; and prevention.

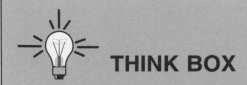

THINK BOX

Money. Is it all about money? The NHS is the world's largest remaining nationalised industry. Yes, I know it's a point I've already made but it's worth making again. By general consensus, nationalised industries are not very efficient. That's why most countries have got shot of them. The problem with the NHS is that it's a much loved institution and no one has come up with a way of breaking up the NHS without being accused of privatising it, or selling it off. Political death.

That's the problem. It's too big and too cumbersome. All of the leading business gurus and high-flying entrepreneurial types will tell you the same thing. So, back to the question of money. Would the NHS manage on less money if it were run in a different way? Would being more business-like mean less taxpayers' hard-earned cash being tipped down the black hole marked 'health'? Is the basic hypothesis of the reform package wrong?

Here's what the plan says about the direction of travel.

1 The NHS will provide a universal service for all based on clinical need, not ability to pay.

Healthcare is a basic human right. Unlike private systems the NHS will not exclude people because of their health status or ability to pay. Access to the NHS will continue to depend upon clinical need, not ability to pay.

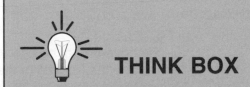

THINK BOX

Right away this starts to get interesting. Where has this phrase 'clinical need' come from? The 1948 NHS Act talks about the 'basis of need', not 'clinical need'. Is the idea of social need excluded?

Make a Note

Is there a conflict between health status and clinical need? Consider a patient suffering from Alzheimer's disease who cannot eat without assistance. Failure to eat will end in starvation and death.

Does assistance with eating become a clinical need or a health need? Is it a social care or a healthcare issue?

2 The NHS will provide a comprehensive range of services.

The NHS will provide access to a comprehensive range of services throughout primary and community healthcare, intermediate care and hospital-based care. The NHS will also provide information services and support to individuals in relation to health promotion, disease prevention, self-care, rehabilitation and after care. The NHS will continue to provide clinically appropriate cost-effective services.

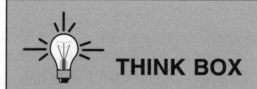

THINK BOX

The NHS Plan seems determined to create more questions than answers.

Make a Note

'Comprehensive', 'clinically appropriate' and 'cost effective'. Are they mutually inclusive or exclusive? Is IVF treatment any of these? Should it be? List other services that are equally difficult to determine under these criteria.

3 The NHS will shape its services around the needs and preferences of individual patients, their families and their carers.

The NHS of the 21st century must be responsive to the needs of different groups and individuals within society, and challenge discrimination on the grounds of age, gender, ethnicity, religion, disability and sexuality. The NHS will treat patients as individuals, with respect for their dignity. Patients and citizens will have a greater say in the NHS, and the provision of services will be centred on patients' needs.

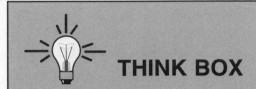

THINK BOX

What does 'having a greater say' mean? We know patients will make rational decisions about core services and rationing, until it's their family that is affected.

Make a Note

Consider where you work and devise a system to involve patients and citizens in planning and shaping the way in which you provide services. Define what contribution you would expect a patient/citizen group to contribute. What could you expect them to contribute over and above your own common sense and your own experiences of using the NHS?

4 The NHS will respond to different needs of different populations.

Health services will continue to be funded nationally, and available to all citizens of the UK. Within this framework, the NHS must also be responsive to the different needs of different populations in the devolved nations and throughout the regions and localities. Efforts will continually be made to reduce unjustified variations and raise standards to achieve a truly National Health Service.

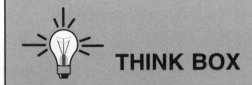

THINK BOX

Mmmm, devolved nations? Is this about the fact that the Welsh Assembly and the Scottish Parliament could decide to offer something different to the English NHS?

Make a Note

Consider the freedom of the Scottish or Welsh executives to make decisions about healthcare in their regions. Rate the likelihood of different decisions evolving into new 'super post code' problems. Where is the best region to live if you need dialysis? Study health deprivation trends. Is equalisation of care a realistic proposition now that we have devolved government? How?

5 The NHS will work continuously to improve quality services and to minimise errors.

The NHS will ensure that services are driven by a cycle of continuous quality improvement. Quality will not just be restricted to the clinical aspects of care, but include quality of life and the entire patient experience. Healthcare organisations and professions will establish ways to identify procedures that should be modified or abandoned and new practices that will lead to improved patient care. All those providing care will work to make it ever safer, and support a culture where we can learn from, and effectively reduce, mistakes. The NHS will continuously improve its efficiency, productivity and performance.

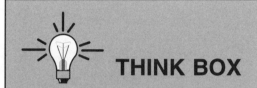

THINK BOX

See that little word at the end, 'productivity'? So, numbers treated are still at the top of the political agenda. And why not? What's the difference between a waiting time and a waiting list if you're in pain? Isn't throughput the issue?

Make a Note

Quality is not to be restricted to clinical aspects of care but include quality of life and the whole patient experience. List the ways in which the patient experience of your services could be improved. Devise ways of finding out what the patient experience is really like.

6 The NHS will support and value its staff.

The strength of the NHS lies in its staff, whose skills, expertise and dedication underpin all that it does. They have the right to be treated with respect and dignity. The NHS will continue to support, recognise, reward and invest in individuals and organisations, providing opportunities for individual staff to progress in their careers and encouraging education, training and personal development. Professionals and organisations will have opportunities and responsibilities to exercise their judgement within the context of nationally agreed policies and standards.

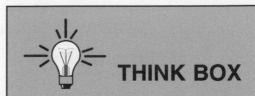

THINK BOX

'. . . exercise judgement within the context of nationally agreed policies and standards.' What does this say about clinical freedom? More freedom or more protocols?

Make a Note

Devise ways to recognise, reward and invest in the people who work with and for you. What assessment tools could you use to discover their training needs? How will training fit both the needs of the individual and the needs of the organisation? Are the two always compatible?

7 Public funds for healthcare will be devoted solely to NHS patients.

The NHS is funded out of public expenditure, primarily by taxation. This is a fair and efficient means for raising funds for healthcare services. Individuals will remain free to spend their own money as they see fit, but public funds will be devoted solely to NHS patients, and not be used to subsidise individuals' privately funded healthcare.

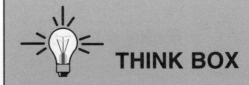

THINK BOX

Doctors and nurses are trained at the taxpayer's expense and are then free to take their skills overseas and eventually into the UK private healthcare sector.

Make a Note

Consider your response to recent press stories about a patient (a hospital manager) suffering from kidney cancer. He was told here in the UK that it was inoperable and he would die. After strenuous efforts searching the Internet, he found a US surgeon willing to operate. The cost was phenomenal and his health authority contributed £30 000. Does item 7

8 The NHS will work together with others to ensure a seamless service for patients.

The health and social care system must be shaped around the needs of the patient, not the other way round. The NHS will develop partnerships and co-operation at all levels of care – between patients, their carers and families and NHS staff; between the health and social care sectors; between different government departments; between the public sector, voluntary organisations and private providers in the provision of NHS services – to ensure a patient-centred service.

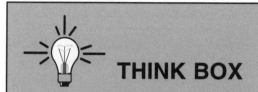

THINK BOX

If we really mean it, how about demolishing social services and handing them over to the NHS to run?

Make a Note

Consider the services you are involved with. Take one sector and devise an approach to teamworking with stakeholders. At what point do the objectives of the individual groups conflict with the needs of the individual, and the model becomes unsustainable?

9 The NHS will help keep people healthy and work to reduce health inequalities.

The NHS will focus efforts on preventing, as well as treating, ill health. Recognising that good health also depends upon social, environmental and economic factors such as deprivation, housing, education and nutrition, the NHS will work with other public services to intervene not just after, but before, ill health occurs. It will work with others to reduce health inequalities.

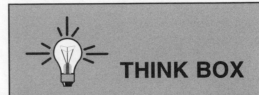

THINK BOX

If we are going to have a real attempt at this, why not start with banning smoking in public?

Make a Note

What are the three greatest causes of social deprivation in the area you work? If you work in a wealthy area don't overlook loneliness and social exclusion through poor mobility – or doesn't that count? What policy initiatives do you need to take to address the causes of the three things on your list?

10 The NHS will respect the confidentiality of individual patients and provide open access to information about services, treatment and performance.

Patient confidentiality will be respected throughout the process of care. The NHS will be open with information about health and healthcare services. It will continue to use information to improve the quality of services for all and to generate new knowledge about future medical benefits. Developments in science such as the new genetics offer important possibilities for disease prevention and treatment in the future. As a national service, the NHS is well-placed to take advantage of the opportunities offered by scientific developments, and will ensure that new technologies are harnessed and developed in the interests of society as a whole and available to all on the basis of need.

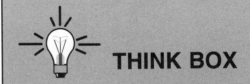

THINK BOX

Is this just 'motherhood and apple pie', or does it come close to a mission statement about the NHS's approach to modern technology? Doesn't it ignore the ethical and moral labyrinth that genetics is going to tangle us up in?

Make a Note

A BMA spokesman is on record as saying that the public will be confused and won't understand comparative hospital outcome data and it will not take enough account of complex case mix variations. Consider a specialty or a service you are involved with and devise a way of making complex outcome information meaningful to patients.

Oh, and don't forget the money

Here's what the extra cash looks like – a 35% increase, in real terms, over four years:

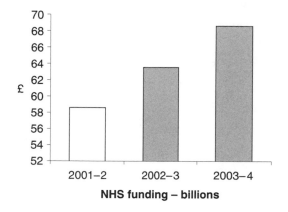

UK spending on healthcare has consistently lagged behind other developed countries. Here are some facts to commit to memory and trot out at meetings to look like you know something – ho, ho!

- Since 1960, Organisation for Economic Co-operation and Development (OECD) countries have on average increased health spending per capita by 5.5% in real terms, compared with only 3.6% in the UK.
- Between 1979–97 the average annual increase in government spending on health was just 2.9%.
- Real terms funding in England has veered between 0% and over 6% a year.
- England has fewer hospital beds per head of population, compared with most other health systems.
- In the NHS there are 1.8 practising doctors per 1000 people, compared with an EU average of 3.1 per 1000.
- One-third of the buildings used by the NHS today were built before the NHS was even created.
- The backlog of maintenance in the NHS now stands at £3.1 billion.
- In 1995, there were approx 360 heart bypass operations per million of the UK population, half of that, for example, in the Netherlands.

. . . and just for the record, here are some data you might like to turn into a PowerPoint slide to impress everyone.

Total expenditure on health as a percentage of GDP (1975 to 1997):

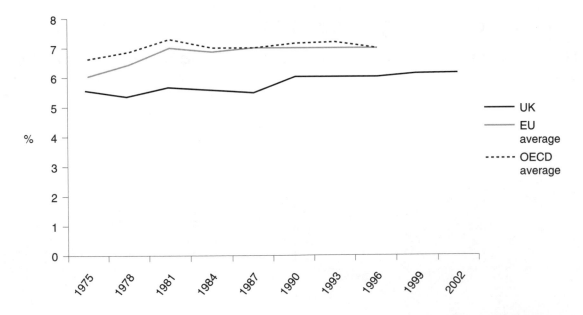

Source: OECD

However, our life expectancy doesn't seem to suffer – funny, eh? We seem to do very well, even if the NHS isn't full of money!

Life expectancy at birth in 1996:

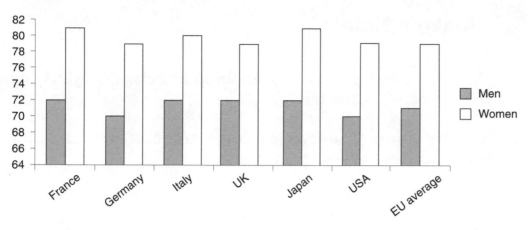

Source: OECD

Perhaps health services have less to do with health than we thought?

Whatever all that means the PM certainly surprised the Treasury, the NHS and most of the cabinet when interviewed by Sir David Frost:

'. . . over time, we aim to bring it [NHS funding] up to the EU average.'

Here's a question for him – but you might like to answer it too . . .

Why?

Sure, any extra money for the NHS is welcome and you'll always find me at the front of the queue. But what's so important about European averages? Who says that is the correct amount of cash for the NHS? Europe is a widely diverse group of nation states with geographical, wealth and educational differences. There are differences in climate, life-style and attitudes. There are different approaches to family, masculinity, femininity and work. There are cultural and religious differences. All of these impact on health. And, European health systems vary greatly in cost and outcomes.

Health is the consequence of wealth, education, social circumstances and job prospects. So why is the European average the Holy Grail for UK healthcare spending?

Make a Note

Make the case for European average health spend being the right amount of money for the UK healthcare system.

Isn't the right answer – however much it takes to keep us all healthy, perhaps it's less than the European average!

Money with strings

There had to be a catch, didn't there? Here it is:

'. . . we offered the nation and those in the NHS a deal. We would spend this money if, but only if, we also changed the chronic system failures of the NHS. Money had to be accompanied by modernisation, investment and by reform. For the first time in decades we had to stop debating resources and start debating how we used them to best effect.'

Here's another interesting bit:

'. . . we have looked at alternative systems and rejected them . . . to make employers and workers pay for healthcare as in France or Germany . . . are all recipes for an unfair system and too great a burden on British families and businesses.'

So much for the European average theory!

The Secretary of State for Health, Alan Milburn, does finally get a few words. Here's what he thinks of the NHS. Do you agree?

Yup, recognise that as part of what's wrong where I work

No, not true at all

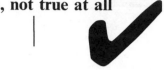

- Not sufficiently designed around the convenience and concerns of the patient.
- Provides many patients with a good and reliable service.
- Not responsive enough.
- Patients have to wait too long for treatment.
- Records get lost.
- Wards are not clean.
- Standards are too variable.
- Old-fashioned demarcations between staff.
- Restricted opening and operating times.
- Outdated systems.
- Unnecessarily complex procedures.
- Lack of training.
- A culture where the convenience of the patient can come a poor second to the convenience of the system.

 ## Make a Note

Consider any one of the 13 points that Alan Milburn makes – the one that you most identify with. Devise an action plan to remedy the situation for you and your colleagues or the staff you are responsible for.

Before you get terminally depressed with all this, take a break and think how good you are!

On a typical day in the NHS:

- almost a million people visit their family doctor
- 130 000 go to the dentist for a check up
- 33 000 people get the care they need in accident and emergency
- 8000 people are carried by NHS ambulances
- 1.5 million prescriptions are dispensed
- 2000 babies are delivered
- 25 000 operations are carried out including 320 heart operations and 125 kidney operations
- 30 000 people receive a free eye test
- district nurses make 100 000 visits.

Do you feel better? There's more. . .

On a typical day in the NHS, there are:

- 90 000 doctors
- 300 000 nurses
- 150 000 healthcare assistants
- 22 000 midwives
- 13 500 radiographers
- 15 000 occupational therapists
- 7500 opticians
- 10 000 health visitors
- 6500 paramedics
- 90 000 porters, cleaners and other support staff
- 11 000 pharmacists
- 19 000 physiotherapists
- 24 000 managers
- 105 000 practice staff in GP surgeries.

Rip this page out and pin it to the notice board or stick it to the fridge door with one of those funny magnet things. Next time you're in a group of people moaning about the NHS, give them a copy.

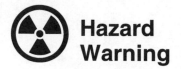

Hazard
Warning

Beware! If the group of moaners have been reading the NHS Plan, they might know there's a huge gap between the best and the rest within the NHS.

- Rates of hip replacement for those aged over 65 vary from 1.5 per 1000 head of population in Doncaster to over 4 per 1000 in Devon.
- Some hospitals carry out almost 100% of cataract removal operations as day cases, others less than 10%.
- For many surgical specialties the top 25% of hospitals get nearly double the output from their consultants as the bottom 25%.
- In the worst hospitals cancelled operations are running at 5%. The best ones have cancellation rates close to zero.
- Often the poorest services are in the poorest areas with the poorest results.

Make a Note

Find out your area rates for cataract removal and hip operations.
Consider the reasons for your fantastically good performance, or not!

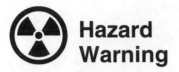

Hazard Warning

The moaners might even tell you about their last trip to a hospital and how many times they had to give their details to a member of staff. Here's a typical list:

	The same where you work?	
	No	Yes
• GP		
• practice nurse		
• hospital booking clerk		
• hospital nurse		
• care assistant		
• therapist		
• junior doctor		
• consultant		

Why change?

Well, that's not the question. We know why, it's the how that's the problem. One of the key problems, sighted in the Plan, is the lack of incentives in the system to improve performance.

Make a Note

List the ways the private sector works to improve performance. What incentives do they have? What carrots and what sticks? How many of the private sector management tools could be employed in the NHS?

. . . in case you're not sure, here's how it works in the NHS:

- consultant contracts provide a flat salary structure plus rewards for those who build up strong academic reputations and a large private practice
- GP fees and allowances are related to the number of patients registered with them and insufficiently to the services provided and the quality
- GPs are not rewarded to take on additional work to make services more responsive and accessible to patients and to relieve pressures on hospitals
- there are few rewards for working in the poorest areas where primary care is at its worst.

In fact, just about everything that could be wrong with an incentive scheme is wrong with the NHS. Indeed, a hospital which manages to treat all its patients within nine or 12 months rather than 18, may be told that 'over performance' means it has been getting too much money and can manage with less next year. By contrast, hospitals with long waiting lists and times may be rewarded with extra money to bail them out, even though the root of the problem may be poor ways of working rather than any lack of funding.

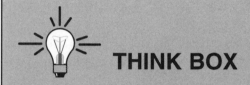 **THINK BOX**

Does the NHS bail out failure rather than reward success? Isn't it often the case that an under performing hospital is just a victim of a poor capitation formulae?

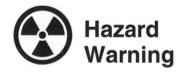 **Hazard Warning**

Before you arrive at a conclusion bear in mind that on one day in September 1999, 5500 patients aged 75 and over were ready to be discharged but were still in an acute hospital bed:

- 23% awaiting assessment
- 17% waiting for social services funding to go to a care home
- 25% trying to find the right care home
- 6% waiting for the right homecare package to be organised
- almost three quarters were not getting the care they needed because of poor co-ordination between the NHS and other agencies.

Make a Note

Find out what the situation was in your area in September last year.

Is it all social services' fault?

Social services come in for all kinds of stick. They are criticised for acting too quickly, they are criticised for acting too slowly. They are criticised for funding the wrong things and not funding the right things. You must have done something really bad in a previous life to end up working in social services.

But is that really true? Doesn't the poor relationship between health and social services often stem from the fact that health and social services are two separate, independent organisations, with their own rules and approach, both trying to serve the needs of the same customer? . . . sorry, client or patient, whichever you prefer.

Make a Note

Consider the working relationships you have with social services. How would you characterise them. How would they characterise the relationship they have with you? Do you see each other as unresponsive, or perhaps trapped in a complex system that doesn't let you do what you know is needed or right? Does the partnership work well? If so, is it because, or in spite, of the rules? Arrange to meet informally with some social services colleagues and discuss the issues of partnership.

There's a lot that needs changing, isn't there? Does any of this ring a bell?

- Lack of time and support to learn from others about what works.
- Isolation of individual hospitals and primary care services from one another slows the spread of good practice.
- Good and bad practice is stuck in their own ghettos.
- Performance inhibited by lack of reliable information for clinicians, managers and patients.
- Data on clinical, primary care and hospital performance are only just starting to be published.
- The NHS is historically poor at linking related pieces of information, such as prescription to diagnosis, so the results can be collated and used nationally to inform practice, monitor and learn from errors.

It gets worse!

- Most GPs are only now compiling registers of their patients at risk from heart disease.
- Managers cannot compare costs of services or establish how different staff and organisations are delivering different results for patients.
- Data are generalised and are too poor to help creative commissioning and the allocation of resources.
- There is no systematic way of independently assessing NHS performance.

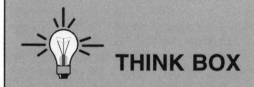

THINK BOX

Strange all this, isn't it? Didn't some wise soul say we shouldn't worry about the cost and complexity of the NHS because costs would fall as the health of the nation improved! What went wrong?

What are the alternatives?

How about private medical insurance? Often touted as a viable alternative to a tax-funded system, it seems to be at the heart of Tory policy. Here's what the NHS Plan thinks about private medical cover.

Private insurance

In 1990 the previous government introduced tax relief on private medical insurance for the over 60s. Despite annual public spending of £140 million on these incentives the numbers of subscribers to private medical insurance rose by only about 50 000 in seven years. This 1.6% increase therefore had only a marginal effect on the NHS.

More recent experience from Australia confirms this analysis. Three years of experimenting with increasingly costly public subsidies – totalling £1 billion – appears to have merely stopped a long-term decline in the coverage of private health insurance. These subsidies have mainly benefited those already with insurance and so far may have added much more to public spending than to private funding.

Second, using public money to pay for tax incentives diverts funds from the public healthcare system. The cost of providing tax relief to those who already have private health insurance would be significantly over £500 million – the so-called deadweight cost. Unless taxes were to rise or spending in another area of government were to fall, that would mean the NHS budget being reduced by the same amount.

Third, it's misleading to presume that incentives for people to 'go private' saves the public sector money. This is because the saving to the NHS is likely to be outweighed by the 'deadweight' costs of subsidising those who already have private medical insurance.

A recent report from the Institute for Fiscal Studies concluded that 'It's extremely unlikely that the cost of any such subsidy to private medical insurance would be less than the NHS expenditure saved'. In other words, switching public funding from NHS expenditure to spending on tax reliefs could reduce health spending overall.

Fourth, the development of genetic testing will affect the coverage and cost of voluntary private health insurance. Healthcare risks will become more transparent. As a result, premiums will rise to reflect high-risk subscribers' likely claims, reducing the affordability of cover, and lower risk subscribers will drop out. The combined effect will be to erode the risk pool on which private health insurance depends.

Fifth, whether or not the introduction of tax relief increased the overall volume of healthcare, it would certainly inflate its costs:

Labour costs: currently there is no surplus of doctors and nurses in our country. The previous government considered the introduction of tax relief in 1988. As Nigel Lawson, the then Chancellor of the Exchequer, concluded 'If we simply boost demand, for example by tax concessions to the private sector, without improving supply, the result would not be so much a growth in private healthcare, but higher prices'.

Fragmentation: the more fragmented commissioning of healthcare becomes, the more prices would be likely to rise. In the USA, for example, pharmaceutical prices are on average 75% higher than in Britain. This is at least in part due to the fragmentation of healthcare purchasing.

Administration: administrative costs would rise significantly. The costs of management and administration are much higher under private insurance because of the bureaucracy needed to assess risk, set premiums, design complex benefit schedules and review, pay or refuse claims. These raised costs impact on hospital budgets. Administrative costs in America are up to 15% higher than in Canada, largely because of the cost of insurance processing.

The implication is that much of any increase in private medical insurance in Britain would go in administrative costs with no direct benefits to patients.

Equity

Private medical insurance is inequitable. Subsidising private health insurance will use taxpayers' funds to expand two-tier access to healthcare, reducing equitable access to needed care. The costs of private health insurance per individual are substantial. For a 65-year old private health insurance costs around 50% more than the equivalent NHS cost.

Private medical insurance shifts the burden of paying for healthcare from the healthy, young and wealthy to the unhealthy, old and poor. The cost of private health insurance rises the older and sicker the person – indeed beyond a certain age, and with chronic conditions, it's virtually impossible to get private insurance cover. Tax relief for private health insurance by definition is regressive. It offers public subsidies to the better off and is meaningless for the worst off.

This view is borne out by findings from a large scale research study in the early 1990s which looked at the costs across income classes of healthcare in Europe and America. It concluded that 'the two countries with predominately private financing systems – Switzerland and the US – have the most regressive structures overall . . . The group of countries with the next most regressive systems are the countries operating the so-called social insurance model, . . . countries which rely . . . mainly on tax finance . . . have the least regressive financing systems'.

This looks like a pretty comprehensive demolition of private insurance systems – can you make the alternative case?

Make a Note

List four reasons why private medical insurance is a good alternative to a state funded system. Why four? Dunno, try five or six if you can think of them!

You could make a start with the fact that a state system is inherently inefficient because there is no competition. Private systems have competition which is a driver for quality and efficiency.

How about the other old chestnut – charges?

Back to the plan:

roponents of patient charges argue that new charges should be introduced for a range of health services to encourage responsible use of resources and raise more revenue for the NHS.

Where charges are high they generally reduce service use across the board. The most thorough study of charges and cost-sharing, the RAND Health Insurance Experiment (a randomised trial undertaken in the USA in the 1970s) found that charges led to less use of preventative care.

The available evidence suggests that they are also likely to discourage use of necessary services. As the World Health Organization recently noted: 'The use of co-payments has the effect of rationing the use of a specific intervention but does not have the effect of rationalising its demand by consumers'.

Lower use and delayed access to healthcare services, especially preventive services, may divert demand to more costly parts of the system and may result in higher healthcare costs in the longer term.

It's sometimes suggested that these undesirable behavioural effects can be avoided by setting new user charges at a low level. Where charges are low they raise very little cash, which may be off-set by administrative and collection costs. For example, in 1992 New Zealand introduced charges for the use of hospital beds. The difficulty of collecting the charges from patients led to their rapid abolition. Equally, in countries such as France that make widespread use of charges, many individuals take out supplementary insurance just to pay them, thus defeating the object of introducing the charges at all.

Charges are inequitable in two important respects. First, new charges increase the proportion of funding from the unhealthy, old and poor compared with the healthy, young and wealthy. In particular, high charges risk worsening access to healthcare by the poor. As the World Heath Organization report – which assessed the United Kingdom as having one of the fairest systems in the world for funding healthcare – concludes: 'Fairness of financial risk protection requires the highest possible degree of separation between contributions and utilisation'.

Second, exempting low income families from user charges can create inequities for those just above the threshold. High user charges with exemptions can create disincentives to earning and working through the imposition of high marginal tax rates. Some European countries do make more use of user charges than Britain. For example, in parts of Sweden in 1996 there were charges for seeing a GP of about £10 per visit and for seeing a consultant about £20 per consultant.

They are able to do so in large part because they tend to compensate people indirectly through the social security benefit system. Even so, in Sweden there is evidence that user charges for visiting primary care doctors have discouraged people from seeking treatment.

Continental social insurance
There are those who advocate maintaining the current role of public funding but shifting wholesale to a social insurance-based model. This is similar to both the German and French healthcare systems. The proponents of this model argue that it leads to larger shares of national income going to healthcare.

Social insurance systems involve payments from individuals just like tax-financed systems. In the French and German social insurance systems, costs fall predominantly on the employer and employee and so fewer people contribute. An outline estimate from 1997 is that a wholesale switch to funding the NHS predominantly from national insurance contributions would cost an extra £1000 per employee using the French model of public healthcare funding, and about £700 per employee per year using the German model, without any increase in the total amount of resources going to the NHS. These calculations adjust for the different levels of expenditure in the three countries, i.e. French and German expenditures are assumed to be reduced to current British levels. At 2003–4 levels of funding, additional costs would be the equivalent of £1500 per worker per year using the French model and £1000 using the German model, again with no addition to currently planned NHS funding.

Continental social insurance models are less efficient in several respects. First, because of the design of the social insurance systems in continental Europe, it's not clear that all of the extra spending is spent efficiently. Cost control under European social insurance systems has been weak because payers have acted as financial intermediaries within the healthcare system but have not played a role in scrutinising the performance, efficiency and effectiveness of the system itself. In the words of the German Head of the Federal Association of General Sick Funds: 'Germany pays for a luxury car but gets a medium-range car in return' and 'if we don't look out, our medium-range car will soon be without brakes and wheels'.

The French system, despite patient choice, is wasteful in the use of many of its resources. Over prescribing is common. At only 3%, generic prescribing rates are far lower than the 60% found in Britain. To tackle these inefficiencies France and Germany are turning to healthcare management mechanisms which have been in operation in Britain for many years, such as a GP referral-based system of primary care.

Second, in recent years fiscal policy and competitiveness considerations have forced all governments to subject social insurance systems to increasingly tight regulation. By placing caps on contribution rates or expenditure, the national governments in Germany and France now effectively determine overall expenditure under their social insurance systems rather than the social insurance partners. In other words, levels of health funding are increasingly unrelated to the system of raising finance and increasingly related to how much the economy can afford and the level of priority placed on health spending by the public.

Somehow I don't think the Gods of Whitehall like that idea either! But should we just dismiss charges?

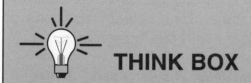

THINK BOX

Making a case for charges is easy but you are always left with the question, what do you do for folk who can't afford to pay? The answer is, you relieve them of having to pay rather like we exempt certain people from prescription charges. This is where the idea starts to fall over. Something like 80% of all prescriptions are free. So if we used the same categories to exempt people from hospital charges, only 20% would pay and the money raised would probably be outweighed by the cost of exemption and collection. Looks like the Gods of Whitehall might be right.

Make a Note

Can you make a case for charges?

And then there was the even older chestnut – rationing

The solution sometimes suggested is that the NHS should be restricted or 'rationed' to a defined core of individual conditions or treatments. There are several problems with this suggestion.

First, advocates of this position usually have great difficulty specifying what they would rule out. The sort of treatments that commonly feature include varicose veins, wisdom teeth extraction or cosmetic procedures. The problem is that these sort of services account for less than 0.5% of the NHS budget, and are not major cost-drivers for the future. Instead, the vast majority of spending – and spending increases – go on childbirth, elderly care, and major conditions such as cancer, heart disease, and mental health problems.

The second major problem is that different patients under different circumstances often derive differing benefits from the same treatment. The NHS is not a system under which each patient only gets a fixed 'ration' of healthcare, regardless of their personal need and circumstances. The fact that a patient has previously been treated for one condition will not of itself prevent her or him from being treated for subsequent conditions. If however 'rationing' merely means that it has never and will never be possible in practice to provide all the healthcare theoretically possible, then it's true of every healthcare system in the world.

The issue is not *whether* the NHS – just like every other public or private health service – has to set priorities and make choices. The issue is *how* those choices are made. Under the NHS, treatment is based on people's ability to benefit. We are in a period of significant expansion of health service resources. The issue is how to improve decisions about how those expanded resources are used. We can no longer leave to chance decisions about how treatment is provided, how demand is managed, and how costs are driven.

National Service Frameworks and the broad priorities set out in this NHS Plan provide the context. The National Institute for Clinical Excellence will help the NHS to focus its growing resources on those interventions and treatments that will best improve people's health. By pointing out which treatments are less clinically cost-effective, it will help free up financial headroom for faster uptake of more appropriate and clinically cost-effective interventions. This is the right way to set priorities: not a crudely rationed core service.

So, the solution isn't rationing! Government is hoping that the National Institute for Clinical Excellence (NICE) will sort out the treatments that are worth paying for and dump the ones that don't work or do not represent value for money.

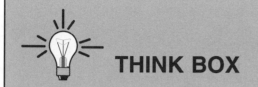

THINK BOX

That's OK up to a point. But there are two problems. The first is that NICE is a small organisation – presently with 28 staff and a budget of just over £10 million (soon to be increased). This makes it way too small to cope with the expectations of Ministers, the Department of Health and the service in general. Don't forget, every time they say no to a drug, the drug manufacturer appeals, wriggles, screams blue murder and eggs the press on. It's difficult to see whether NICE is waving or drowning! Government has made NICE a lynch pin of its policies – they will have to think again about its size and capacity. And second? Much more difficult. What happens when NICE runs out of things to say 'No' to? 'Yes' costs money, doesn't it?

The bricks and mortar

Here's the problem. In the last 10 years average bed stays, across all hospital specialties, have fallen from an average of just over 10 days to just under five days. Bear in mind that this is an average across **all** specialties.

The effects of medical technology, new drugs, faster recovery times from operations, new anaesthetics and modern surgical techniques are bringing the average down, even as you read this page!

Nevertheless, the NHS Plan calls for:

- 7000 extra beds
- and 100 hospital projects.

This conclusion is based on the outcome of the National Beds Enquiry, a consultation exercise 'inviting members of the public and professionals to tell the government what pattern of services the NHS should provide in the future'.

Bear in mind that hospital consultants like to build up their empires with a nice few beds – 'thank you'. And a bit of spare capacity in the system makes bed management a bit easier – 'thank you'. Trade unions like more beds because it means more staff – 'thank you'. Did they ask the right people and have we got the right answer? They asked:

- PCGs
- health authorities
- trusts
- Royal Colleges
- doctors
- nurses
- other health service professionals
- academics
- local councils
- community health councils
- unions
- charities
- private companies
- representative organisations.

 Make a Note

Think about the impact of technology on a specialty where you work or one that interests you. Will improvements to that service depend on more beds and more hospitals? Are we building more problems for ourselves? Consider telemedicine, hospital-at-home services, improved drug therapies, better co-ordinated discharge . . .

The Plan also calls for:

- 5000 extra intermediate care beds, some in community or cottage hospitals others in specially designated wards in acute hospitals; some will be in purpose built new facilities or in redesigned private nursing homes
- 1700 extra non-residential intermediate care places
- a 30% increase in adult critical care beds over the next three years.

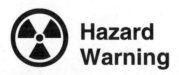 **Hazard Warning**

Didn't we close down cottage hospitals? Didn't we have trouble with night cover, resuscitation and emergency events? Didn't we decide they were too expensive to maintain, heat, light, insure and look after, and had an average bed unit cost twice the price of a night in the Hilton Hotel on Park Lane, London?

Make a Note

Consider planning a capital development. What calculations could you take into account to make a case for more beds? Bear in mind the likely impact of technology on the approach to treatments, the potential for day case treatment and patient preferences to be treated nearer to, or where possible at, home.

Technology or not, here's what's going to happen. Great news for the building industry but I'm not so sure about the taxpayer and the NHS:

- nine new hospital schemes given the go ahead in 2001 – worth £1.3 billion
- nine new hospital schemes given the go ahead in 2002 – worth £1 billion
- 100 new hospital schemes in total between 2000 and 2010
- 20 diagnostic and treatment centres developed by 2004.

Funding for many of the developments is through PFI schemes and up to £600 million will be released through a one-off auction of empty and surplus NHS property.

THINK BOX

Does the NHS have to own its property? A large slice of the NHS estate will be owned by the private sector anyway. Given the uncertainties that technology and medical advances create for deciding just how much real estate the NHS does need, wouldn't it be a better idea to take the responsibility for property away from Trusts and put it all into a Plc company (shall we call it 'Sick Brick Plc')? This would produce a massive flotation and make loadsa money available for the NHS to spend on things much more useful than buildings. The company would benefit from a steady revenue stream from the rents the NHS would pay, from disposal of unwanted assets and development of buildings and capital projects we do need.

Looks like it's not such a daft idea. Primary care might get there first.

Enter the latest NHS acronym – 'NHS LIFT', otherwise known as the NHS Local Improvement Finance Trust. In some parts of the country, mainly in inner city locations, primary care premises are poor. At the heart of the difficulty is the fact that primary care is also poor. The simple truth is that middle class doctors often don't want to work in run-down difficult neighbourhoods. Thankfully, some do but a lot don't!

LIFT will improve primary care premises in England. Up to £1 billion will be invested in primary care facilities and some 3000 family doctor premises will be refurbished.

The aim is to bring together, under one roof, all the primary care services patients might need. A one-stop shop for:

- primary and community services
- social services
- GPs
- dentists
- opticians
- health visitors
- pharmacists
- social workers.

The aim is to build, or develop, 500 of these by 2004.

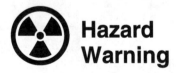 **Hazard Warning**

By when? 2004! That's 48 months away! Doesn't that mean building 10 a month? How long will it take to design the thing, acquire the land, obtain planning consent from the local authority, go out to tender for the building contract, build the building and make a date in the PM's diary to come and open it? 500 in four years sounds like some going to me . . . pity the project manager who gets lumbered with this job!

Make a Note

Consider a project to create a one-stop primary care facility in your area. What is a realistic, fast track timetable?

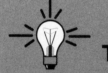

THINK BOX

By the way, how long before the Treasury says 'Hold it, let's save some money and put all this lot together and call it a hospital'?

Pulling services together comes close to the vertically integrated care model now being developed in parts of the US. They've given up on trying to get primary care going. Now they put all the services under one roof – primary and secondary care.

OK, we've got the buildings, what are we going to put in them?
Answer: loadsa nice new kit. £300 million's worth to be precise:

- 50 new magnetic resonance imaging (MRI) cancer scanners
- 200 new CT cancer scanners – 150 replacements, plus 50 additional
- 80 new liquid cytology units to improve cervical cancer screening
- 45 new linear accelerators – 20 replacements, plus 25 additional
- 3000 new automated defibrillators in public places to help save the lives of the one in five people whose heart attacks occur in a public place
- 450 new and replacement haemodialysis stations.

Make a Note

Consider the staffing implications of the influx of new equipment. Select an item of equipment that could be used where you work. Work out the staffing implications and the revenue implications for the wage bill. Then consider the consequences for subsequent treatment – the impact on capacity to treat, staffing and recruitment.

Also consider the impact of developments in diagnostic technology. Do we really want this traditional sounding kit? Isn't there anything new on the horizon?

We've got the buildings and the kit: can we keep it clean?

Hospitals should be the cleanest places on God's earth. Why is it then that around 1500 people die every year from hospital-acquired infections? Some say that the deterioration in standards of cleanliness is all down to compulsory competitive tendering – fluff busters at the cheapest price. Is that true? Doesn't tendering out cleaning services provide an opportunity to draw up some tight service level agreements?

Like it or not there's going to be a national 'Clean Up the NHS' campaign, with £30 million ready to fund it.

Here's the checklist:

- all patient areas
- visitor toilets
- outpatients and accident and emergency units
- chairs, linen, pillows, furniture, floor coverings and blinds – those beyond repair will be replaced.

Make a Note

This is serious stuff! National standards for cleanliness are to form part of National Service Frameworks and a hit squad is likely to descend upon you and check out for 'spick and spanness'! Are your current arrangements up to it?

Ward sisters and nurses are expected to take a lead in ensuring wards are properly cleaned – what will be their likely training requirements to take on this role? Consider what adjustments you may need to make to your cleaning contract. Draw up an inspection protocol to arrive at these new levels of cleanliness. Evaluate your current cleaning arrangements and decide whether or not they are robust enough to achieve the new levels required.

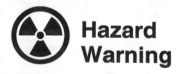 **Hazard Warning**

Does your current contract allow for mid-term modifications? Will you be able to negotiate new standards and working practices?

Cleanliness Tsar needed!!

A member of the Board is to be given personal responsibility for monitoring hospital cleanliness, and will report to the Board following regular check ups.

 Make a Note

Develop inspection protocols for a Board member to undertake this new duty.

What are the qualities needed to carry out the role? A cleanliness freak who looks under all the beds? A realist who realises that hospitals are busy places and get scruffy from time to time? Mmmm, could be tricky!

Devise a format to report to the Board. Remember, the key to reporting is that it should be consistent (so that trends can be identified), inclusive and presented in such a way that other Board members can understand it.

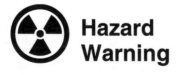 **Hazard Warning**

A few hospitals have already been checked up on by Department of Health fluff busters. Apparently, they've reported the results to the Secretary of State for Health but not to the Trust bosses.

Trust CEOs have been given self-assessment forms and the results of the two are compared. Obviously evaluating perceptions. One man's fluff is another man's insulation, no doubt!

Done the fluff, what about the food?

As Michael Caine might say 'Do you know, the NHS provides over 300 million meals each year at a cost of £500 million?' No? Well, like the man said, not many people know that!

Wait, how many meals and for how much? 300 million into 500 million makes that about £1.60 a meal! No wonder some of it tastes like %$&*! What can you expect to get for £1.60 a meal? On that basis NHS food must be a miracle.

 Make a Note

Find out the cost per meal where you work and go and pat the Kitchen King on the back!

As a result of the NHS Plan, by 2001:

- a 24-hour NHS catering service with a new NHS menu, designed by leading chefs. It will cover continental breakfast, cold drinks and snacks at mid-morning and in the afternoon, light lunchtime meals and an improved two course evening dinner – this will be a minimum standard for all hospitals
- a national franchise for NHS catering will be examined to ensure that hospital food is provided by organisations with a national reputation for high quality and customer satisfaction
- half of all hospitals will have new 'ward housekeepers' in place by 2004 to ensure that the quality, presentation and quantity of meals meets patients' needs
- patients, particularly elderly people, are able to eat the meals on offer
- round-the-clock dieticians to advise and check on nutritional values in hospital food.

Make a Note

Don't dismiss this, meal standards are set to become part of the Performance Assessment Framework and there will be unannounced inspections of the quality of hospital food.

Patients' views are to be sought on the quality and availability of food.

Devise a patient questionnaire to capture their views on catering standards, as part of an ongoing measurement of patient satisfaction.

Bedside televisions and telephones

Here's what the NHS Plan has to say on the subject:

'In an age of cable and digital TV, with over half the population owning mobile phones, people increasingly expect to have access to these services wherever they are. It's no longer acceptable for patients to have to wait for a nurse to wheel a trolley to their bed or have to stand in a draughty corridor if they want to make a call.'

There, I couldn't have put it better myself!

So, what are you going to do about it? Some of the more enlightened hospitals have done the patients a favour and also done themselves a favour into the bargain. They have a nice little earner from a contract with a private company to install bedside TVs and phones. They can make calls at discounted rates and watch videos. One of the channels is dedicated to hospital use for the showing of programmes to help patients prepare for their operation or for explanation of aspects of their treatment.

The Gods of Whitehall seem to like all this and intend to let a major national contract deliver the service, NHS-wide, by 2004.

Make a Note

How many beds do you have that could be linked to a bedside TV/phone service? More importantly, what procedures would you feature on the hospital channel? Is there a risk that patients watching the video alone, could be frightened or put off?

Select a procedure you are familiar with and consider what the content of such a movie might be and how it would best be presented.

All this technology has brought a rush of blood to the head! Take a look at this shopping list:

- electronic booking of appointments for patient treatment by 2005
- access to electronic personal medical records for patients by 2004
- by 2004, 75% of hospitals and 50% of primary and community trusts will have implemented electronic patient record systems
- feasibility study on effectiveness of smart cards for patients allowing easier access to health records
- electronic prescribing of medicines by 2004 including repeat prescriptions
- all GP practices will be connected to NHSnet by 2002.

Why is the NHS such a basket case when it comes to the management of information by the use of technology? Most NHS staff have more computing power in their children's bedrooms than they do at their office desk.

The only reform the NHS really needs is to get the whole NHS on-line and working to reasonable industry comparable IT standards.

The disaggregation of the NHS during the Thatcher years gave Trusts a much needed dose of freedom, but it also meant that strategic purchasing of IT infrastructure was next to impossible. Everyone doing their own thing produced an electronic Tower of Babel. No one was able to talk to anyone but themselves.

In fairness, even though those reforms started as short a time ago as 1990, in the intervening years there has been an explosion in IT capacity and facility that no one could have foreseen.

The benefits of the electronic patient record are almost boundless but beware! Their successful development has defeated almost everyone, including the Americans. Yes, the home of all things 'techie' is still arguing over the best way to capture data and store it. A 2005 target is ambitious . . . very ambitious.

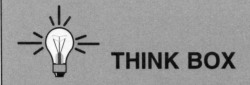

THINK BOX

Electronic patient records should make a huge difference to the efficiency of the NHS. However, think about this – you've applied for a job and it's yours subject to a medical. The HR person says to you 'We don't do a physical medical, we just download your EPR, so if you would give me your NHS smart card for a moment, I'll go and do it now'.

Are you comfortable with that?

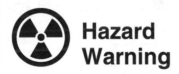

Hazard Warning

The crown copyright software for the standard NHS payroll system, which sorts out the wages and salaries of over 750 000 NHS employees, is more than 25 years old. The Department of Health has started a national procurement process to replace it. This is the good news. The bad news is, when did the NHS last get an IT procurement right! Hang on to your wages – ho, ho!

Make a Note

Consider how a decent IT network would change the life of a nurse on a ward. Think about ordering tests, referring patients, booking appointments, accessing the National Electronic Library for Health to access state-of-the-art information on latest treatments and best practice. In fact, the sort of capacity that airline staff and travel agents take for granted.

List the facilities a nurse might look for in the design of such a system. Take account of items such as touchscreen *vs* keyboard access, screen design and password thresholds.

OK, we've got the buildings and the kit – how about the people?

The NHS Plan is full of good ideas. In truth, few of them are really new. Most of them are already working somewhere buried deep in the NHS! Nevertheless, none of it – good idea, pinched idea, any idea – is any good without the people to make it work.

The NHS is way behind – take a look at the situation regarding doctors.

Practising doctors (density/1000 population) in 1996:

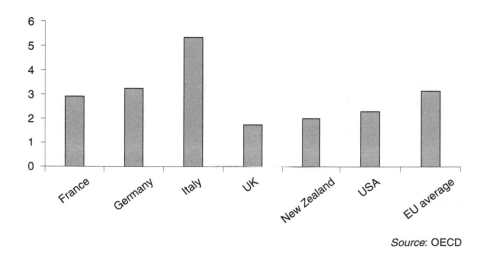

Source: OECD

Everyone is working like beavers. How's the morale over at your place? Feel cherished, loved and valued, or worn out, exploited and fed up?

Make a Note

The morale of an organisation is integral to its performance. Often overlooked as a management lever and usually ignored, staff morale can compensate for all sorts of organisational shortcomings. It's often argued that morale in the NHS is poor. However, given the low working environment base most staff endure, isn't it the case that if morale wasn't high the NHS would have collapsed years ago? Or am I confusing morale with commitment?

Devise some key indicators to define, measure and monitor the morale of the staff where you work.

We all know it takes years to train doctors and nurses, but here's the plan. Between now and 2004 there will be:

- 7500 more consultants
- 2000 more general practitioners
- 20 000 more nurses
- 6500 more therapists and other health professionals
- 1000 more medical school places (on top of the 1100 already announced).

> There are 15 000 vacant nursing posts in England – 5000 in London alone.
>
> What's it like over at your place

Now, it's true that the BMA (signatory to this plan!) is already quibbling about the number of training places and new doctors there're going to be. But let's take a look at the figures on face value. That's close to 36 000 new people joining the NHS at the rate of 750 a month over four years. Mmmm . . .

What's the staffing situation over at your place?

Make a Note

Here are some things to sort out.

- List areas of staff shortage.
- Do these shortages reflect the national picture or is there something unusual about where you are?
- What has been tried to recruit new staff?
- And what hasn't?
- Can you recruit from overseas? Is that ethical? Should we be pinching staff from other healthcare systems that may need their people even more than we do?
- Would a workplace nursery help?
- Have you got one, is it full, is it any good? How do you know?

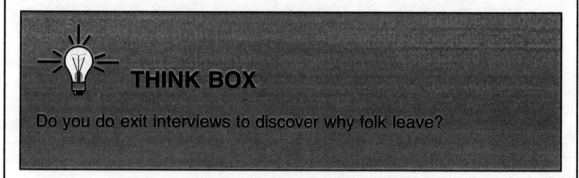

THINK BOX

Do you do exit interviews to discover why folk leave?

- Are shift patterns flexible and family friendly?

Here's what the Gods of Whitehall are going to do to help:

- increase throughput from training
- modernise pay structures and increase earnings
- improve the working lives of staff
- recruite more staff from abroad.

Is it possible?

By 2004, on current plans, government expects more than 45 000 new nurses and midwives to come out of training, and over 13 000 therapists and other health professionals. Plus, further year-on-year increases in the number of training places available for all health professionals.

So, stand by to be amazed and by 2004 expect:

- 5500 more midwives and health visitors being trained each year
- 4450 more therapists and other key professional staff being trained
- 1000 more specialist registrars – the key feeder grade for consultants, targeting key specialties
- 450 more doctors training for general practice.

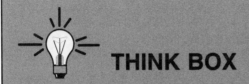

THINK BOX

We all know that the key to reform of the NHS is in recruitment and retention. Attracting the right people of the right quality is increasingly difficult. . . the world of work has changed.

Once, for a young female school leaver the only jobs worth having were in teaching or nursing. All that has changed. Today, a graduate can choose a job with a company car, a good salary and with the prospect of travel and advancement. Or they can become a nurse and not ever earn enough to own a car or pay a mortgage, run the risk of being assaulted and have their social life totally screwed up by shift work!

Too cruel? Maybe, but the point is that nursing, doctoring and all the other professions the NHS depends on, are in competition for recruits. The job market is open like never before.

Make a Note

Prepare a workforce study to take into account service improvements and developments, and the impact they will have on existing staffing levels and the shortages and skills gap they will create.

Consider your recruitment strategy.

Is it just about pay?

For the last two years pay awards recommended by the independent pay review bodies have been implemented in full. Since 1997, nurses have had a 15% pay rise. There has been agreement, in principle, on a new system of intensity payments for consultants to reflect increasing workloads, and a new contract for doctors in training has been negotiated to give more rewards to those working most intensively and doing the most anti-social hours. The government has agreed an above-inflation pay rise for staff outside the Review Body, for three years.

Will it make a difference?

The need to respond to local conditions and the local labour market is as important as having a national strategy. Rejoining schemes and plans to hit labour shortages can only be achieved if employers have local flexibility.

The pay flexibility allowed under the NHS and Community Care Act 1990 allows Trusts greater freedom to recruit and retain locally, with local contracts of employment. For most hospitals, local contracts were too difficult and staff-side organisations resisted them. Some Trusts were more successful than others.

 Make a Note

The government is considering a Market Forces Supplement to deal with some of the local issues.

Consider how you would use such a supplement. Take into account such factors as accommodation costs, rejoining incentives, childcare facilities (including child minders) and other key local issues.

Is it just about money?

Anyone who says they don't work for the money is either a liar or very rich! Of course money plays its part but there's more to a job than wages, and the government seems to have cottoned on to this. They've invented a new Improving Working Lives initiative, which means that employers must demonstrate that they are:

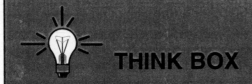

Yup, we're doing all that good stuff, now

Better start work on sorting some of this out

- investing in training and development
- tackling discrimination and harassment
- improving diversity
- applying zero tolerance on violence against staff
- reducing workplace accidents
- reducing sickness absenteeism
- providing better occupational health

THINK BOX

You may think you've got this already cracked but the really tricky areas of discrimination and harassment are difficult to establish, and even more difficult to measure. Few people will admit to being discriminated against and few like to admit any kind of harassment. Creating an open environment, where there are systems and opportunities for people to express their concerns is where it all starts.

Make a Note

Reducing workplace accidents can save the organisation money and the staff a lot of grief. Assemble all the records for accidents that have taken place in the last year where you work.

Carry out a risk analysis. What are the trends? Do some accidents repeat themselves? What is the most common cause of accidents and mishaps?

Consider the policy and training steps you need to take to reduce accidents.

Design a system to measure and record accidents and spot trends early on.

New stuff to cope with:

- a new Performance Framework for Human Resources is due for publication
- . . . and by April 2003, the framework will be incorporated into the overall Performance Assessment Framework
- all NHS employers will be assessed against performance targets and the new Improving Working Lives standard
- all NHS employers are expected to be accredited as putting the Improving Working Lives standard into practice – counselling services, conducting annual attitude surveys, asking relevant questions and acting on the key messages.

Make a Note

Draft a survey to assess staff attitude in connection with the Improving Working Lives initiative. How can you stop the exercise becoming a wish list?

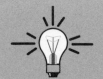

THINK BOX

Have you noticed the number of times the phrase 'national frameworks' is starting to appear? Do you see the emergence of an NHS based on the US Health Management Organisation model? HMOs sit at the centre of the healthcare system and manage by a series of targets, protocols and frameworks developed at the centre. These are turned into management tools by using the data to compare one organisation with another. Simple, eh? And smart too . . .

SECTION 3

Education, education, education . . .

That's a familiar phrase. For the NHS translate it into training, training, training . . .

There's loadsa money coming down the pipeline that is earmarked for training. Some of it is for new initiatives (which will need development and planning) and some for extending existing initiatives.

- £25 000 for every NHS Trust will be provided immediately for tangible, practical improvements in the working environment for staff – to be spent as staff themselves want (whether on providing a face lift to staff rooms or improving other basic facilities) based on responses to the local annual staff survey or other means of staff involvement.

- £6 million in 2001/02 rising to £8m in 2003/04 for extension of occupational health services (already a requirement in hospitals and community trusts) to GPs and their staff. Standards of occupational health services for NHS staff will be included in the Improving Working Lives standard.

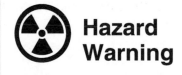 **Hazard Warning**

Be sure to develop robust management tools to determine what staff want this money spent on. Consider brainstorming, face-to-face meetings, questionnaires and suggestion schemes. Remember, it's easy for a vocal minority to hijack these types of initiatives. Consider how your plan will result in fairness and equity for all staff.

You know you've got it right when you can demonstrate:

Done it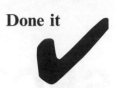

- commitment to more flexible working conditions
- challenges to traditional working patterns
- staff have more control over their own time
- team-based employee-led rostering
- annual hours arrangements
- childcare support
- reduced hours options
- flexi-time
- career support
- career breaks
- flexible retirement
- staff involved in the design and development
  of better working practices and in decisions
  which will affect their working lives.

 Take a break and let's give this some thought. There's more . . .

- expand NHS sponsored and on-site nursery provision (an additional £30m to be invested by 2004)
- by 2004 there will be provision for on-site nurseries at around 100 hospitals, provided at an average subsidy of £30 per place per week

and

- every NHS Trust to have a childcare co-ordinator to be the parent's advocate and adviser (also available to PCGs and PCTs)
- co-ordinate the provision of nursery places and a network of secure provision for school-aged children, drawing on after-school clubs, local childminding networks and holiday play schemes to meet local needs
- a requirement for the provision of on-site nursery and childcare facilities will be built into all plans for new NHS hospitals.

Make a Note

Childcare co-ordinator? Not easy. Create a job description for such a post. Remember, there are huge sensitivities concerning people working with children.

Training for everyone

The NHS is used to the concept of continuous professional development and postgraduate training. However, the NHS Plan opens the door for training opportunities for all staff. There's a new pocket of money, £140 million by 2003/04, to ensure that all professional staff are supported in keeping their skills up to date and to provide access to learning for all NHS staff without a professional qualification.

Make a Note

Develop a skills and learning assessment of staff without a professional qualification. Consider how to find out what their needs are and how their training could bring tangible benefits to where you work.

SECTION 4

New systems

The NHS Plan envisages some new ways of working. Since its inception in 1948 the NHS has been centrally accountable. Each year the Treasury allocates, and Parliament votes, funding to the NHS. It is through Parliament that the Secretary of State for Health is accountable for the money that is spent and the performance of the NHS.

The difficulty is, however, in running and being accountable for an organisation with over 840 000 staff, and a network of hospitals, clinics and units that reaches into every part of England.

Anxious to reassure MPs, at the inception of the NHS, that it could be run from Whitehall, Nye Bevan used the famous phrase 'when a nurse drops a bedpan in Tonypandy, the noise will be heard in Whitehall'. Nice idea but the wrong management message. And, anyway, with respect to the great man, it can't be done.

You'll be pleased to know that the NHS Plan actually confesses:

> **. . . the NHS cannot be run from Whitehall.**

Now, there's an admission that's worth framing! Top-down management tends to stifle innovation but a big sprawling organisation like the NHS needs some tight rules to stop gung-ho enthusiasts disappearing off the management scale and bone idle wasters hiding in the undergrowth. What's the answer?

Well, it has defeated just about every government who has tried to reform the NHS since 1948. Let's see if this lot are likely to be any luckier!

A new delivery model

The Plan proposes a new relationship between centre, region and locality. The NHS is an organisation glued together by a bond of trust between staff and patient – what some have called 'principled motivation'.

Oh yes! Nice phrase, right out of the Plan! It's all about words . . .

A new word to play with

The reformed NHS will be run on the principle of 'subsidiarity'. Where have you heard that one before?

Isn't it something to do with our relationship with the European Union? Don't the folks who are nervous about admitting that one day we'll be run from Brussels, use the phrase? What does it mean? Here's how the *Collins English Dictionary* defines 'subsidiarity':

> 'the principle of devolving decisions to the lowest practical level.'

Here's what the Plan says:

'The principle of subsidiarity will apply. So the centre will set standards, monitor performance, put in place a proper system of inspection, provide back up to assist modernisation of the service and, where necessary, correct failure.'

There's more:

'Intervention will be in inverse proportion to success – a system of earned autonomy. The centre will not try and take every last decision. There will be progressively less central control and progressively more devolution as standards improve and modernisation takes hold.'

Let's look at that in a bit more detail and pick out a few key words:

- set standards
- monitor
- inspection
- correct failure
- earned autonomy.

Interesting what you can do with words, isn't it!

If you can be bothered to go back five or six pages, you'll find one of those Think Boxes with the lightbulb icon. To save you the enormous effort of turning pages, here it is again:

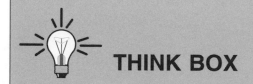

THINK BOX

Have you noticed the number of times the phrase 'national frameworks' is starting to appear? Do you see the emergence of an NHS based on the US Health Management Organisation model? HMOs sit at the centre of the healthcare system and manage by a series of targets, protocols and frameworks that are developed at the centre. These are turned into management tools by using the data to compare one organisation with another. Simple, eh? And smart too . . .

It looks like we are on the right track. Indeed, the NHS Plan admits it. Here's what it says in paragraph 6.8:

6.8 In future the Department of Health's role will involve championing the interests of patients by applying both pressure and support. It will do this by:

- *setting the priorities* for improving the nation's health, and allocating funding to local health services working with patients and the professions to *develop national standards of care*
- putting in place a robust management and support framework to deliver those standards
- *monitoring and holding the NHS to account* so that patients know how well the NHS is performing
- *intervening* on behalf of patients only where NHS organisations are failing to deliver proper standards of care

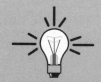

THINK BOX

This is very close to the US HMO model. The question is, will the development of frameworks, protocols, standards and targets be more or less likely to promote innovation and preserve clinical freedom? Perhaps the best question is, does it matter if it doesn't? If the service ends up faster, safer, modern and more dependable, isn't that what counts? *(Modern, Dependable – where have I heard that before? Ed)*

Let's look back at the italicised bits again and do a bit of joined-up-ness:

'setting the priorities; develop national standards of care; monitoring and holding the NHS to account; intervening . . . where NHS organisations . . . failing to deliver proper standards.'

See what I mean? This is looking like a very different NHS! And there's a lot more of it to come.

The NHS Plan sets out the main national priorities and the standards will take three forms.

1 National standards for key conditions and diseases through National Service Frameworks (NSFs). NSFs have already been produced covering mental health and coronary heart disease, and in the autumn will be followed by the National Cancer Plan. A NSF for older people's services is due to be published in autumn 2000 and one for diabetes in 2001.

2 Clear guidance on the best treatments and interventions from NICE. This year NICE is due to undertake 23 appraisals and issue 10 sets of guidelines. As part of the Plan, the work programme of NICE will be increased. It will carry out 50% more appraisals and produce 50% more guidelines. To enable it to carry out this extra work, NICE's budget will be increased by £2 million.

3 A number of other national targets, including: shorter waiting times; the quality of care and facilities for people whilst they are in hospital; new services to help people remain independent; and efficiency.

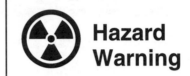

Hazard Warning

These five service frameworks between them cover services that account for around *half* of total NHS spending.

Expect to see further NSFs developed on a rolling basis over the period of the Plan. Good practice saves money, doesn't it?

Redesigning services, to borrow a phrase from the management gurus, is all very well, but what about the customers? Earlier in this book we dealt with the customer/patient 'who's what and which is who' issue. But it's worth revisiting here. No point redesigning if we end up with something that's no better for patients.

What is 'better for patients'? How do we know? If all else fails we could always ask them! Planning the pathway or route that a patient takes from start to finish to see how it could be made easier and swifter – every step, from the moment a patient arrives at the GP's surgery, up to and including when they are discharged – is not a new trick but it's a trick that is not done often enough.

If we can:

- remove unnecessary stages of care
- arrange for tests and treatments to be done on a one-stop, day case basis
- and decide which professional should carry out which functions,

we end up with the beginnings of a standard guideline or protocol for a condition.

Where this has been done the impact has been dramatic and has resulted in improved services for patients. It has also resulted in improved productivity, made the task of caring for patients easier for staff and in many cases it has released resources to spend on other services.

Care pathways were pioneered in the mid-1990s but have been very slow to be adopted by the whole of the NHS.

 Make a Note

Select a condition you are familiar with. Plot the patient's route through the service, from the first appearance of symptoms through diagnosis, treatment and return to function. If you can, involve a group of patients in the exercise to gain a full understanding of the pathway they took. Look for variations and develop a care pathway that would have improved the experience for them all.

If you think this isn't worth bothering with, I've news for you. If you don't do it yourself, you're going to get some help!

Enter the Modernisation Agency – more top–down stuff . . .

A new Modernisation Agency is coming to help you whose purpose is to help local clinicians and managers redesign local services around the needs and convenience of patients.

It will take over:

- the existing National Patients' Action Team
- the Primary Care Development Team
- the 'Collaborative Programmes'
- the clinical governance support unit
- the NHS Leadership Centre
- the Beacon Programme
- the NHS Annual Awards programmes.

Do you want to go and work for them? You might be able to as the staff will mostly be drawn from the NHS on secondment, and be based within the regional offices.

This is all very top–down. So, to make it bottom–up, guess what? Yup, you've got it – Trusts are expected to set up teams to implement this new patient-centred approach in their own organisation.

 Make a Note

The aim of all this 'modernisation' is to create a more personalised care at the heart of the service. Consider your organisation's response to this initiative. Design a team to enable local implementation and evaluation of services for patient friendliness.

Consider the size of the team and the skills needed to 'bring something to the party'.

Make a Note

The Modernisation Agency's initial work programme will look at projects to cut waits and streamline care for:

- orthopaedic
- dermatology
- ear, nose and throat treatment.

Select one group and design an audit to identify ways of streamlining care. Speak with all the care givers along the pathway and talk with patients who have travelled that route. Look for differences in expectations, assumptions and experiences.

Even more top–down stuff. The Department of Health is cross-dressing as an HMO!

A Performance Assessment Framework (PAF) has already been introduced that covers the six key areas of NHS performance:

1 health improvement
2 fair access to services
3 effective and appropriate delivery of healthcare
4 outcomes from healthcare
5 efficient use of resources
6 high-quality experience for patients and carers

and each year tables are published showing how each health authority has performed against the measures in each category. There are going to be five changes to the way performance standards are set and information is collected and published. Pay attention, this means you.

1 From April 2001, a version of the PAF will be compiled that specifically applies to all NHS Trusts and PCTs providing community services, including specific information on patients' views, quality of care, the workforce and efficiency.

2 NICE, CHI, the Audit Commission, patients' organisations and the Royal Colleges will develop proposals for improved measures.

3 Responsibility for the annual publication of PAF results will be transferred to CHI who will work in association with the Audit Commission.

4 By April 2001, every GP practice and PCG/T must have in place systems to monitor referral rates from every GP practice, to match the information currently available on GP prescribing.

5 New efficiency targets will be set based on levels of service already being achieved by the best Trusts around the country.

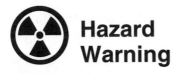 **Hazard Warning**

So the rest will have to reach the standards of the best. This is not for fun, I think they really mean it! This is likely to be a very big challenge for some units. Think about the issues that can skew hospital performance. Social demography, the 'wellness' of the communities they serve, staff availability, cash allocations – shall I go on?

And let us not forget that the information is to be published. You can bet your life that the local press will ignore the 50 things you are really good at, and major on the two things you didn't do so well.

This starts to be a public relations nightmare as well as an organisational challenge. Name and Shine or Name and Shame.

The inspector calls

Well you couldn't have all that comparative stuff without an inspection, could you? Here's what the NHS Plan has to say on the subject.

- The NHS, like other public services, needs to be subject to independent scrutiny. Local people have the right to know how effective their local health services are. In addition, inspection helps identify all that is good about an organisation as well as highlighting problems that need to be addressed.
- The Commission for Health Improvement will quality-assure the care of NHS hospitals as well as community and primary care services.
- The Commission for Health Improvement, with the support of the Audit Commission, will inspect every NHS organisation every four years.

- To support this expanded role for the Commission for Health Improvement, its current size is set to double over the next few years.

It also says . . .

- The government will also continue to use its powers to send the Commission into those Trusts where there are serious and urgent concerns about clinical practice or patient safety.

Here's what the boss of the Commission, Peter Homa, said:

> 'CHI is not Off-Doc, Off-Sick, or NASTY.'

I think Peter must have been on leave on the 28 October 1999 – look what the Secretary of State for Health said:

'CHI signifies our refusal to tolerate second best anywhere in the NHS.'

And here's what the Prime Minister said on the same day:

'a standards watchdog . . . Rooting out bad practice . . . Examining the quality of care from the patient's perspective.'

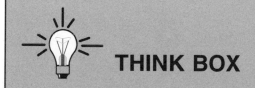 **THINK BOX**

Isn't there a bit of a gap between the boss from the Commission and Number 10? Peter Homa is a seasoned, experienced and very good NHS manager who is, rightly, endeavouring to make CHI a learning experience, developing people and sharing good practice.

Do the politicians see CHI in a different light? The language is about 'inspection' and 'rooting-out'. All very different in tone.

Whilst this book was being written seven NHS Trusts were named and shamed for lagging behind in the waiting list sweepstakes. The CEO of one of the hospitals only found out he was on the list when his press officer told him he'd seen it in the press. Another knew he had a problem, had actually asked for help and yet was still shoved on to the name and shame list. Punitive or supportive? Your call!

And another thing . . .

CHI plans 100 inspections every year. That's at least 100 people if they go on their own, and there's no one left in the office to answer the telephone! We know that NHS managers never go anywhere alone and inspectors hunt in packs. Assume a 48-week year and half a dozen inspectors for each job and a support staff back at the ranch, and you get some idea just how big the Commission is going to be.

Finally, where will the inspectors come from? Well, that's CHI's biggest weakness. They will be managers, on secondment, from other parts of the NHS!

Now, let's remember for a moment how nasty everyone has been about self-inspection, investigation and regulation in the police service, the railways, the nuclear industry and the medical and nursing professions. Well, the managers are going to do it too. CHI is self-regulation.

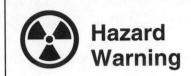 **Hazard Warning**

We know how difficult it has been for clinicians to blow the whistle on poor practice. How difficult might it be for an ambitious NHS manager to be critical of colleagues? After all, one day they may meet again on an interview panel, looking for the next job. Self-regulation sucks!

SECTION 5

That's enough stick, what about the carrots?

Now comes a new guru phrase – 'earned autonomy'.

Depending on how you do against the Performance Assessment Framework, all NHS organisations (health authorities, NHS Trusts, PCGs, PCTs and HAZs) will for the first time annually and publicly be classified as 'green', 'yellow' or 'red'.

Otherwise known as 'management by traffic light'.

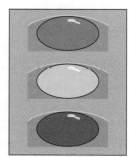

Criteria will be set nationally but assessment will be by regional offices with independent verification by the Commission for Health Improvement.

Here's how it works.

- **Green** organisations will be meeting all core national targets and will score in the top 25% of organisations on the Performance Assessment Framework, taking account of 'value added'.
- **Yellow** organisations will be meeting all or most national core targets, but will not be in the top 25% of Performance Assessment Framework performance.
- **Red** organisations will be those who are failing to meet a number of the core national targets.

So red status will result from poor absolute standards of performance, and you can expect the boot to be put in.

Green status reflects both outstanding absolute performance against core national targets and relative performance against the wider Performance Assessment Framework measures, serving as an incentive for continuous improvement on the part of all organisations. The 25% threshold for green status will be reviewed periodically. It's not just how well you are doing.

The potential for a good hospital to be found in the middle of a dodgy health authority area is recognised in the appraisals system. However, as many aspects of performance span organisations across a health community, the criteria for traffic lights will explicitly include how well they work in partnership with others, and how well the local 'health economy' as a whole is performing on key shared objectives.

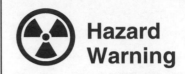

Hazard Warning

So be nice to CHI when they descend on you. Why? How well or badly you do will probably be understood where you work, but score a yellow or a red and you'll spend the next six months sorting out the local press, and the six months after that explaining why any bright, new consultant, nurse or manager would want to work in a basket case hospital.

The moral of the story is 'be nice to everyone and all play together like good girls and boys!'

If you end up in the green, what can you expect?

- Automatic access to the National Performance Fund (of which, more later) and discretionary capital funds without having to bid.
- Lighter touch monitoring by the regional offices.
- Less frequent monitoring by CHI.
- Greater freedom to decide the local organisation of services.
- Being used as beacons or exemplars for the Modernisation Agency.
- Having the ability to take over persistent failure red light organisations.

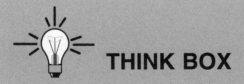

THINK BOX

Be honest, which of these rewards drives you wild with desire? What's in it for the staff? Aren't all of these 'rewards' the sort of thing that might make managers' lives a bit easier? But what's in it for the average nurse up to his/her armpits in muck and bullets on a geriatric admissions ward?

In addition, green health authorities will be 'licensed' to take over delegated regional office performance management functions in relation to the local NHS, including NHS Trusts. Over time, within a national framework, this would allow the progressive devolution of performance management and strategic development from the Department of Health, and a streamlining of the 'intermediate' tier.

Something tells me that a management guru is likely to take the view that shuffling jobs around does not lead to greater efficiency.

What about some cash?

From April 2001, your vulgar attachment to filthy lucre will be recognised. The government will introduce a National Health Performance Fund building up to £500m a year by 2003/04.

The bad news is that the fund will be held and distributed regionally. The good news is that it creates an opportunity to get your hands on your share of a health authority's average allocation of £5 million.

Make a Note

How many NHS units are there in your health authority area? Take a stab at guessing how many of them are likely to end up in the 'green' zone. Divide the number of 'greenies' into £5 million. How much have you got? Is it worth the effort?

A word of caution before you celebrate – the yellows and the reds might be able to sneak a few quid out of the fund too.

'Red' organisations will have their share of the performance fund held by the new Modernisation Agency. They will get their fair share of extra funds but it will come with strings attached.

So, can you:

Yup!

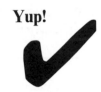

- reduce waiting times?
- introduce booked admissions?
- redesign waiting out of the system?
- improve the quality of care?
- adopt local referral protocols based on national clinical guidelines?
- wear your underpants over your trousers and leap tall buildings in a single stride?

. . . because that's the sort of thing that will keep you in the green!

Work in a PCG or PCT? Add this lot and become a greenie:

Yup!

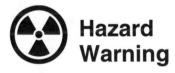

- ensure referrals to hospital are appropriate and help achieve shorter waiting times
- develop joint working between PCGs, NHS Trusts and social services to achieve improvements in rehabilitation facilities for older people.

⚛ **Hazard Warning**

'Ensure referrals to hospital are appropriate and help achieve shorter waiting times.' Mmmm, couldn't this mean delaying a referral in order to produce the impression of a shorter wait?

Make a Note

You won't become a 'greenie' without a team effort and it's important that the rewards on offer reward the team. Consider how the rewards might be used. Include:

- money to buy new equipment or upgrade facilities to improve patient care
- improved facilities and amenities for staff
- non-consolidated cash incentives for individuals and teams.

Develop an approach to determine how the team would want to spend the cash. Avoid being hijacked by the department that shouts the loudest!

Why bother with this? Because the Gods of Whitehall intend to pilot the use of team bonuses in a number of NHS Trusts from next year. See, it must be worth the price of this book to discover that!

And when it all goes pear shaped? Here's what you must hope never happens to your place . . .

Failing organisations will be subject to a rising scale of intervention reflecting the seriousness and persistence of their problems. 'Red' organisations – those whose performance calls for 'special measures' – will receive expert external advice, support and, where necessary, intervention.

'Red' organisations on special measures will be legally directed to produce a detailed recovery plan, which includes milestones and measures to put right concerns reported by the Commission for Health Improvement. The recovery plan will have to be agreed with, and will be overseen by, regional offices.

In the case of persistent clinical failure in a 'red light' organisation, NHS Trusts will be able to draw on the limited number of medical consultants that the Modernisation Agency will employ on a retainer basis in each region. They will be geographically mobile, and will be seconded in to provide clinical leadership and, where appropriate, direct patient care in Trusts with enduring performance problems.

As a last resort, those 'red' organisations that exceptionally fail to respond to special measures and meet their recovery plan will be put under the control of a new replacement senior executive, non-executive and clinical team. Clinicians and managers from 'green' organisations could be deployed for this purpose. Alternatively, expressions of interest could be invited from elsewhere, and subject to a tender from an approved list. Trusts could be merged or large Trusts split up into smaller or different clinical configurations where appropriate.

Where persistent failure is identified in a PCG or PCT, responsibility for leading primary care in the area affected could be transferred to a neighbouring PCG or PCT on either a temporary or permanent basis.

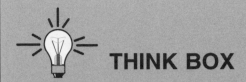

THINK BOX

Consider the recent crop of bad news headlines about the performance of certain parts of the NHS. How much of that would have been avoided with 'traffic light' management? Consider too the effect on staff of a hostile take over of a failing Trust.

This approach to leveraging performance moves us away from the reforms of 1990 where it was expected that GP referrals would simply not be made to an underperforming department or unit. The problem is that most areas are not served by enough hospitals to make real choice an option. How will patients take being referred to a 'red light' hospital and treated by parachuted-in managers and doctors?

Once again the real problem doesn't seem to lay in sorting out a hospital, the problem is sorting out the press and public relations.

How are you doing?

Expect a little light bedtime reading. An independent annual report on progress in implementing the NHS Plan will be published and a Modernisation Board, composed of health professionals, patient and citizen representatives and frontline managers drawn from 'green light' NHS organisations, will be busy writing it.

The new chief executive of the NHS will have three jobs – public health, the NHS and social services – and will report to the Modernisation Board and be accountable for delivering the NHS Plan. Fancy a new job?

Under the Plan, the Secretary of State will shed some responsibilities.

- Decisions on the take up and use of drugs and treatments will be made by NICE.
- The Commission for Health Improvement is to inspect every part of the health service.
- The appointment of non-executive directors of Trusts and health authorities will pass to a new NHS Appointments Commission.
- The Commissioners will replace the current posts of Regional Chairs.
- Decisions on the outcome of major health service reorganisations will in

future be based on the recommendations of a new National Independent Panel which will advise on contested major changes.

• Hearing of consultants' appeals against dismissals will in future be dealt with locally rather than by the Secretary of State.

 So, what's the boss going to do all day!

Speaking at a healthcare conference, a nurse famously said that when he grew old he didn't care if the hand that wiped his bottom was a health hand or a social services hand, just as long as it got wiped!

The divisions that exist between the NHS and social services are well known and well documented. They are organisations that are poles apart in managerially, financially and organisationally trying to look after the same customer.

If patients are to receive the best care, then the old divisions between health and social care need to be overcome.

Health and social service relationships seem patchy. In some parts of the NHS the services work well together, in other parts the story is grim.

 ## Make a Note

Consider the NHS/social service relationship – they are divided by:

• different funding streams
• different managerial structures
• social services are accountable to elected members of a local authority, the NHS is not
• definitions are not the same.

What other differences account for the difficulties in working relationships?

Evaluate the working relationship you have with your social services. What is the biggest impediment?

The Health Act 1999 has made some changes to working relationships and has ended some of the legal obstacles to joint working. The major changes are:

- **pooled budgets**: allowing health and social services to combine resources into a single dedicated budget to fund a wide range of care services
- **lead commissioning**: either the local authority or the health authority/PCG takes the lead in commissioning services on behalf of both bodies
- **integrated providers**: local authorities and health authorities merge their services to deliver a one-stop package of care.

 Make a Note

Evaluate a joint health and social service project. Consider tools to measure the success of the joint work. How could it be improved?

The NHS Plan promises a £900 million investment in intermediate care services, where pressure is at its greatest.

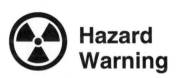 **Hazard Warning**

New incentive schemes for social services to promote partnership working come with strings! Strings called 'Joint Best Value' inspections of health and social care organisations.

 Make a Note

Make a serious effort to find out about best value evaluations – they are like competitive tendering with knobs on, complete with bear traps!

If you boys and girls won't play together nicely, the government is going to make you!

The problem is that while Health Act schemes cover budgets of over £200 million, only a small minority of patients are benefiting. In the future government intends to make it a requirement for these powers to be used in all parts of the country rather than just some.

 Make a Note

The result will be a new relationship between health and social care which has the potential to radically redesign the care system.

Working with social services won't be a novelty – it will be a necessity. Find out how social services work. Visit their offices and understand their working methods. Take time to sit in the public gallery at a meeting of the social services committee in your area. The more you can find out about social services the more you'll understand them and the easier it will be to work with them.

Make a Note

Consider the benefits to the patient of better joint working. List the service improvements they might expect.

Here are a few to get started:

- a single care plan
- a single key or link worker
- a unified multidisciplinary team
-
-
-
-

. . . how many can you list?

Older people usually suffer the consequences of poor NHS and social services relationships – however, the Plan provides an extra £900 million investment (by 2003/04) in new intermediate care and related services, with the aim of promoting independence and improved quality of care for older people.

The cash also brings some targets – PCGs, PCTs and local authorities will have to put in place the following services:

- **rapid response teams**: made up of nurses, care workers, social workers, therapists and GPs working to provide emergency care for people at home and helping to prevent unnecessary hospital admissions
- **intensive rehabilitation services**: to help older patients regain their health and independence after a stroke or major surgery.

Make a Note

Consider to what extent these services are already provided. If they are provided, what are the workforce implications in extending such services?

If they are not provided, why not? To what extent does the availability of money solve the problem, or are there other issues? If so, what are they?

 ## Make a Note

Consider the types of joint service NHS and social services might offer:

- recuperation facilities
- one-stop health and social services available for the elderly
- integrated home care teams
-
-
-

How many can you list? Feel free to write in the margin!

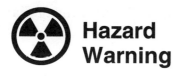 ## Hazard Warning

These changes are fundamentally focused at primary care. Did you know that government expects all PCGs to be PCTs by April 2004? Was that in your plan?

The invisible join

Get ready for a new kid on the block (another new kid!) – the Care Trust. A pretty unimaginative name for an imaginative idea!

Care Trusts will be able to commission and deliver primary and community healthcare as well as social care for older people and other client groups. Social services would be delivered under delegated authority from local councils. Care Trusts will usually be established where there is joint agreement at local level that this model offers the best way to deliver better care services.

First the stick . . .

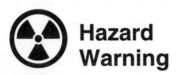

Hazard Warning

Where local health and social care organisations have failed to establish effective joint partnerships – or where inspection or joint reviews have shown that services are failing – the government will have the power to establish integrated arrangements through the new Care Trust scheme. The Commission for Health Improvement, the Audit Commission and the Social Services Inspectorate will use the Best Value system to jointly inspect health and social care organisations to see how well they are implementing these arrangements.

Now the carrot . . .

Local authorities, health authorities, PCGs and PCTs will receive incentive payments to encourage and reward joint working. In the case of health organisations it will be through the National Performance Fund. In social services £50 million a year will be available from April 2002 to reward improved social services joint working arrangements, based on measuring performance from 2001. From April 2003 the fund will rise to £100 million. It will operate as a ring fenced grant and will be focused initially on intermediate care performance.

Make a Note

The two funds will have common criteria. Select initiatives where joint working with social services could have an immediate impact on the care for the elderly in your area.

PCGs will probably have the best opportunities to improve care by working with social services, developing easier-to-access and more convenient-to-use services.

Get ready, the first wave of Care Trusts could be in place next year! Yes, next year and there is a rush to get some key deliverables in place by the next election.

SECTION 6

What about the docs?

By and large, GPs work in a system that has changed little since 1948. Whether the plan delivers more doctors is still the source of a row between the doctors and the DoH, notwithstanding the fact that the BMA is a signatory to the document and is supposed to be all loved up and signed up!

The Plan says:

'Our family doctors are a real source of strength for the NHS. As a result of the changes in this Plan we will have strengthened GP services still further: there will be 2000 more GPs and 450 more GPs in training by 2004. This will just be a start – faster growth of the number of GPs will need to continue beyond 2004.'

The docs say:

'The Plan's promise of an extra 2000 GPs in England is a 7% increase on the current 28 500. This represents an increase of 1.6% a year.'

Dr Hamish Meldrum, joint deputy chairman of the BMA GPs' Committee, said: 'Before the plan was announced we were already getting an extra 0.9% so the real increase is only 0.7% a year. We are now seeing over 70% of training places going to women, who will want time off for their families. We estimate that for every GP who retires we will need to enrol 1.5 or 1.6 GPs to replace them.'

Who's right? Mmmm, difficult call. Dunno. But given this government's reputation for funny numbers, double counting and spin, my money is on the docs. But why is our mate Hamish-the-Doc talking about 'women who will want time off for their families'? Wake up doc, so will men! Think about paternity leave, family friendly policies and the fact that there are more women in the world than men!

Changes for NHS doctors:

- expansion of medical students, specialist registrars, consultants and GPs
- further expansion to follow
- move to new quality-based contracts for GPs
- new arrangements for single-handed practices
- new contract for consultants
- extra rewards for consultants tied to NHS service
- up to 3000 family doctors' premises including 500 new primary care centres will benefit from a £1 billion investment programme by 2004
- GPs will be helped with their continuing professional development through earmarked funds
- NHS occupational health services will be extended to cover family doctors.

So, what are they moaning about?

Here's the key issue. As usual it's a pay and rations issue.

The current GP contract – the 'Red Book' – has often worked well, but it places greater emphasis on the number of patients on a GP's list and the quantity of services provided, rather than the quality of them. Too often it has been an obstacle to GPs who have wanted to develop services tailored to the needs of their own local population.

There is also an assumption that some GPs want to spend at least part of their career as a salaried doctor rather than an independent contractor. Since 1998 an increasing number of GPs have been working to a different type of contract – the Personal Medical Services (PMS) contract – instead of the standard national contract.

PMS pays GPs on the basis of meeting set quality standards and the particular needs of their local population. For example, if an area had a particularly high level of heart disease, the PMS contract could set targets for ensuring that local people at risk are identified and prescribed appropriate treatment.

In some PMS schemes all members of the healthcare team – doctors, nurses and other health professionals – work on a similar contract instead of the traditional arrangement where staff work for a self-employed GP.

PMS also allows GPs, if they choose, to work on a salaried part-time or full-time basis.

Doctors cherish their self-employed status and don't like the idea of being salaried – they certainly don't like the idea of a life full of targets, incentives and goals. Some think they should just get paid on the numbers treated and not on the way their work is targeted.

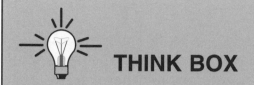

THINK BOX

Government must realise that they get primary care on the cheap. 'Self-employed' means that GPs take care of themselves. They organise their own leave, sort out their office needs, hire staff and manage their businesses. Salaried staff will be looking for company cars, locum cover organised for them and all the other stuff that employees take for granted and the self-employed sort out for themselves.

This is not about the government wanting more salaried doctors, it's all about shaping doctors' work around the needs of their communities. It's about focus, goals and outcomes.

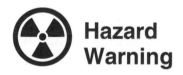

Hazard Warning

Expect a major expansion of PMS contracts. All the current successful pilot schemes will become permanent. By April 2002, expect nearly a third of all GPs to be working to PMS contracts.

A PMS standard core contract cuts bureaucracy and is formed on the basics: delivering key objectives such as access to primary care, NSF standards, quality and clinical governance.

The national 'Red Book' contract will be amended to reflect the emphasis on quality and improved outcomes inherent in the PMS approach. By 2004, both local PMS and national arrangements are set to operate within a single contractual framework.

. . . and single-handed practices?

A certain doctor, whose name I do not have to mention, is in prison following the murder of a number of elderly patients and it's suspected that he committed umpteen more murders than he was charged with. Grim news that has shocked the medical establishment, frightened the public and seems to have forced ministers up a blind alley.

You see, the problem is compounded by the fact that the doctor in question was a so-called single hander, meaning that he worked alone – the implication being that if he had not worked alone the murders would never have taken place. This is of course rubbish. Single handers are committed, popular and work very hard.

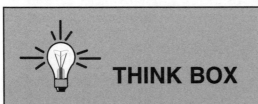

THINK BOX

Who knows what goes on behind the closed door of any doctor's surgery – single hander or not. Time we installed CCTV!

Indeed, they are much less likely to be involved in medical politics, take time out to go to meetings and more likely to form close and trusting relationships with their patients. It does not mean they are more, or less, likely to be the kind of nut-case who murders their patients.

There is no evidence to suggest that single handers give better or worse care, although there is evidence that patients do better when they get to know their doctor well.

The Gods of Whitehall have decided that 'they [single-handers] do not have the ready support from colleagues [that is] enjoyed by GPs in larger practices. The current "Red Book" contract is a particularly poor mechanism for protecting quality standards in these practices'.

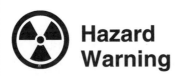 **Hazard Warning**

New contractual quality standards will be introduced for single-handed practices. This will either be done through a negotiated change to the 'Red Book' or, if this proves impossible, a new national PMS contract will be introduced into which all single-handed practices will be transferred by 2004.

In other words, if you don't like it, lump it.

Make a Note

Who do you think a patient would best like to be treated by? A bright young GP in a busy practice, who is interested in being on the PCT Board and keen to develop his/her career, speaking at and attending conferences? As a consequence their patients are often seen by other partners in the practice or by a locum.

Or a single hander who doesn't get involved with the medico-politico rubbish, is up to date, keeps his/her head down and is only interested in looking after patients, their families and carers?

. . . and the hospital doctors?

Local NHS Trusts have had to contribute part of the cost of specialist registrar posts. As a result a large gap exists between the number of specialist registrar posts planned for nationally and the number of posts that have actually been created at local level.

This will now change. From 2002 the government will centrally fund all specialist registrar posts.

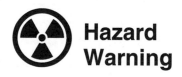

Hazard
Warning

. . . but only on the proviso that agreement can be reached with the medical Royal Colleges. But they have signed up to the plan – not that that seems to be a guarantee of anything!

Let's hope they've negotiated the next bit. There are two options:

1　an expansion in the number of non-consultant career grade doctors, often on Trust-specific contracts, **or**
2　continuing hospital care as a consultant-delivered service.

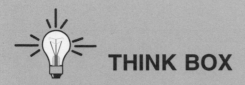

THINK BOX

Which option is best for doctors? Which option is best for Trusts? Which option is best for patients?

The first option would allow the NHS to get more fixed clinical sessions from senior doctors without competing with private practice. In the second option there is a clear career structure and doctors are certain about how they will progress and where contractual obligations to the NHS are unambiguous.

Can we expect to keep recruiting doctors or is it more realistic to recruit technicians who are skilled in one particular treatment and nothing else? Is it realistic to train doctors for 14 years before they become consultants? Is this modern workforce planning or should we be looking at different ways?

The old chestnut about consultants and their right to private practice seems to rumble on. Few have the proper job plans they are supposed to have and managers still seem reluctant to manage the consultant workforce. Even fewer have their performance regularly reviewed.

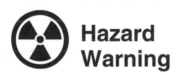

Hazard Warning

A new consultant contract envisages annual appraisal and mandatory job plans so that NHS employers can manage the consultant workforce effectively, thus ensuring the best use of their time and Trust resources. Royal Colleges will be able to advise NHS Trusts on, but not veto, job descriptions for consultant posts. All consultants will have job plans specified by the employer linked to annual appraisal of their work. Don't expect the Colleges to roll over on this one – they may have signed the Plan but not a death warrant!

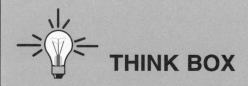

THINK BOX

What are the options? Could the NHS 'buy-out' private practice? This is likely to cost at least £700 million and the NHS would end up in a bidding war with the private sector – not practical. It's a bit like promising to re-nationalise the railways – it would please some parts of the Labour party and give the Treasury a fit. Not surprisingly, the government has backed off on this one.

Instead . . .

At present, the consultants' contract requires them to work an ambiguous 'five to seven' fixed sessions a week. In future, existing consultants will be, by default, contractually required to undertake seven fixed sessions a week, pro rata. Trusts will be able to fund extra, fixed consultant sessions on an as-needed basis, as at present. Assuming this condition and other aspects of the reformed consultant contract are met, existing consultants will continue to undertake private practice in their own time.

And, the Plan says . . .

'A move to a consultant-delivered service means that in future, newly qualified consultants will be contracted to work exclusively for the NHS for (perhaps) the first seven years of their career, providing eight fixed sessions, and more of the service delivery out of hours.'

Note the use of the word 'perhaps'. In fact, newly appointed consultants do not customarily embark on private practice for at least five years. Oh and let's not forget that Peter Hawker, chairman of the BMA Consultants' Committee, told the *Guardian*:

The plan showed a 'profound lack of understanding of the work they [consultants] do'. And their [the government's] only new idea was 'an ill-conceived and vindictive attack on new consultant's freedom to work outside the NHS'.

Guardian 28 July 2000

So, expect a war . . . Yup, I know the BMA is supposed to be signed up to all this. Ho, ho!

What's at stake?

How much do consultants earn in the private sector? Data are hard to come by. However, in their third report the Parliamentary Select Committee on Health produced some numbers.

Assuming consultants do private work when they are not working in the NHS, how often do they work in the NHS? Good question. The Select Committee thought it was a good question too.

Indeed, in their report they actually commented that it was 'extremely surprising that there were no accurate and independent figures showing the average hours worked by the 23 000 NHS consultants'.

The Audit Commission survey suggested that fewer than 70% of consultants were attending 90% of their fixed sessions.

Bad show girls and boys.

NHS consultants' earnings from private practice:

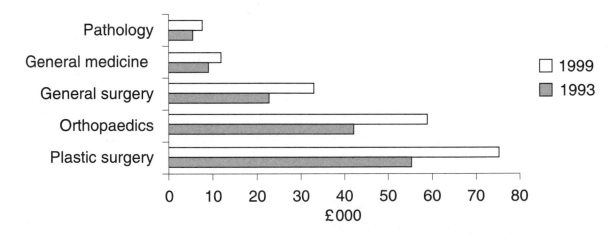

Source: Select Committee

The graph shows average earnings for the years 1993 and 1999. The figures for 1999 are the Select Committee estimates. No wonder they don't want to give it up! A fair few foreign holidays and school fees there!

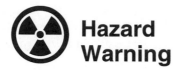

Hazard Warning

Junior doctors don't like the idea of a sub-consultant grade and at the BMA's conference pushed through a motion calling for the resignation of the President of the Royal College of Obstetricians and Gynaecologists who supports the idea – look out for a row. This is not over yet!

And, there's more to upset poor Peter Hawker . . .

The Plan continues:

'In return we plan to increase the financial rewards to newly qualified consultants. Beyond this, the right to undertake private practice will depend on fulfilling job plans and NHS service requirements, including satisfactory appraisals. **If agreement cannot be secured to these changes the government will look to introduce a new specialist grade for newly qualified hospital specialists to secure similar objectives.'**

There's the warning.

Make a Note

What's the future for consultants and their private practice? After a full day's work in the NHS is it safe to work on in the private sector? If a consultant has spent the weekend operating in a private hospital, is it safe for him to come into work on a Monday morning and open up a few NHS patients? How does private practice sit with the requirements of clinical governance?

What about a few carrots?

Consultants can expect bonus payments from the National Performance Fund and a reform of the existing distinction awards and discretionary points schemes.

Together they provided £170 million last year in superannuable bonus payments, ranging from £2500 to £60 460. They will be merged into a single, more graduated scheme with increased funding to enable more awards to be made.

 Make a Note

What should the payments be made for? The Plan says they should be paid to consultants who make the biggest contribution to the delivery and improvement of local health services, and to ensure that bigger rewards go to consultants who make a long-term commitment to the NHS. Do I hear you ask, what about the patients?

Expect explicit criteria for the new single scheme by the end of 2000 and the arrangements to come into force by April 2001. Let's hope Peter Hawker is on the docs negotiating team – this should be fun!

It's a safe bet that the new scheme will be weighted in favour of consultants who are contracted exclusively to the NHS. There will also be special provision for clinical academics (and for the first time academic GPs) and consultants of national and international renown.

Medical Education Standards Board

Who are they? They will replace the separate bodies for general practice (the Joint Committee for Postgraduate Training in General Practice) and hospital specialties (the Specialist Training Authority).

The Board will ensure that 'patient interests and the service needs of the NHS are fully aligned with the development of the curriculum and approval of training programmes'. So now you know!

Fancy being on the Medical Education Standards Board? Membership of the new body will be drawn from the medical profession, and the NHS and the public.

Oh, and then there's the General Medical Council . . .

What can be said about the GMC that hasn't been said already? Useless basket case or struggling with an out of date framework and trying to get its act together? Your call.

They have a consultation document whizzing around the system and if they manage to hang on, they're going to have to be more responsive to patients, faster acting and more transparent.

Think they can do it? More about them later, I'm delighted to say!

That's enough about the docs, what about the others?

SECTION 7

Changes for nurses, midwives, therapists and other NHS staff

'This is not a question of staff working harder. It's about working smarter.'

Snappy, eh? Not the sort of phrase you expect to see in a government publication but it's right there.

 Make a Note

Why do you think it is that in some accident and emergency departments nurses are treating patients with minor injuries and ailments, freeing up doctors' time, delivering shorter waits for treatment and some are not?

In some community clinics teams made up of occupational therapists, district nurses, physiotherapists and social care staff have halved the length of stay for orthopaedic patients, and enabled more frail people to stay at home. It's true, isn't it, that for every example of good practice there are too many examples where change has yet to take place.

List some reasons why the NHS is so slow to cascade good practice.

By 2004, the majority of NHS staff will be working under agreed protocols identifying how common conditions should be handled and which staff can best handle them.

The new NHS Modernisation Agency (remember them?) will lead a major drive to ensure that protocol-based care takes hold throughout the NHS. It will work with NICE, patients, clinicians and managers to develop clear protocols that make the best use of all the talents of NHS staff and which are flexible enough to take account of patients' individual needs. Here's a reminder about what we might have already concluded about protocols, national frameworks and stuff like that:

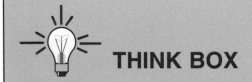

THINK BOX

Have you noticed the number of times the phrase 'national frameworks' is starting to appear? Do you see the emergence of a NHS on the US Health Management Organisation model? HMOs sit at the centre of the healthcare system and manage by a series of targets, protocols and frameworks that are developed at the centre. These are turned into management tools by using the data to compare one organisation with another. Simple, eh? And smart too.

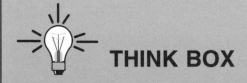

THINK BOX

Will this new approach end the old demarcations? Do demarcations just mark the end of one set of skills and the beginning of another? If all staff become generalists will there be increased dangers for patients? Or will appropriately qualified nurses, midwives and therapists undertaking a wider range of clinical tasks including the right to make and receive referrals, admit and discharge patients, order investigations and diagnostic tests, run clinics and prescribe drugs (which is what is proposed), lead to better care?

As part of this approach, by 2001 around 23 000 nurses will have the right to prescribe a limited range of medicines. That might work out to be around 50 nurses in each Trust.

The introduction of 'Patient Group Directions', enabling nurses and other professionals to supply medicines to patients according to protocols authorised by a doctor and a pharmacist, will mean that by 2004 the majority of nurses should be able to prescribe. That's better!

There is also the little matter of carrying out a wide range of resuscitation procedures, including defibrillation (shouldn't we all be able to do that?). And they are all going to be able to perform minor surgery and outpatient procedures. Remember the old adage 'the more you do, the better you get at doing it'?

And the pharmacist?

Surely the greatest underused resource in the NHS? It's all set to change as they climb out of the canyon between the hairspray and the lipstick. Pharmacists will take on a new role as they shift away from being paid mainly for the dispensing of individual prescriptions towards rewarding overall service. Proposals will be invited for PMS-type schemes that pilot alternative contracts for community pharmacy services, covering medicine management and repeat prescribing.

 Make a Note

List innovations that pharmacists could make to play a bigger role in primary care.

This is all exciting news for staff who are keen to develop their skills but it's important that staff feel confident enough to take on new responsibilities. There's some cash to help you become more confident!

To help people take on these new roles there will be an extra £140 million by 2003/04 to support a major programme of training and development. And no, you can't have it all.

For professional staff there will be investment to support their continuing development. Here's the important bit – the government intends to open discussions with the professions and NHS employers about how to guarantee this commitment. Make sure you have your say!

No professional qualifications? Cheer up, as over the next three years we will guarantee all such staff access either to an individual learning account of £150 a year or dedicated training to NVQ Level Two and Three.

 Make a Note

Consider staff in the roles of healthcare assistants, operating department practitioners, pharmacy technicians and others. What type of training could these staff be offered? Design a skills audit to discover where extra training is needed. What kind of appraisal systems could you use to make sure the best use is made of the money and the individuals get the best out of it?

What about training a few more technicians? Assistant practitioners in radiography, taking on and speeding up breast screening programmes. That's the plan. In industry such a plan would be called 'de-skilling' but you can bet that the NHS will have a less threatening word for it!

Make a Note

Think of other professions that can be de-skilled and think of the impact on waiting times – nurse nephrologists, physician's assistants. But keep it quiet . . .

What will the future of training look like?

For nurse education and training, look no further than the nursing, midwifery and health visiting strategy *Making a Difference.* Not read it? Shame on you, it's riveting! Full of emphasis on improving access and developing practical skills early on in training.

Nurses are set to take on more of the repertoire of doctors . . .

> **Stop Press!**
>
> The RCN is balloting its members on allowing NVQ trained and healthcare assistant staff into the College. About time too!

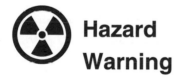 **Hazard Warning**

If nurses are going to do more of what the doctors do, who's going to do what the nurses used to do?

There is a serious question to be asked about the future of nurse training. Quite rightly nurse leaders want nursing to become a profession and nurses to become as professional as possible. They argue that if the nursing community is highly qualified they will then be equipped to take on more senior and demanding roles, and take over some of the work of doctors – prescribing, some procedures, diagnosis and discharge.

As a result, some nurse leaders want nursing to be a graduate entry profession. This would disqualify a whole section of would be nurses who, for a variety of very good reasons, feel unable to enter into university education. Consequently, we would lose the opportunity to employ bright, intelligent, caring people who, with appropriate training, could do the job very well.

A further consideration is the fact that years ago young female school-leavers (and nursing is still a 90% + female occupation) had little choice in the jobs market. Secretarial, nursing and teaching were the available careers. Today, a graduate woman has a world of work choices undreamed of 10 years ago. The work opportunities landscape for women has changed beyond all recognition with careers that provide security, company cars, share options, sensible hours, career breaks, family friendly policies and advancement.

However hard the public sector tries, it will always be on the back foot in the modern jobs market. Is nursing going in the right direction?

If you are a nurse be sure to get a copy of *Making a Difference*. If you are not a nurse, be sure to read a copy. Nursing is pivotal to the NHS workforce and if you're not a nurse, over 300 000 of your colleagues are – so find out what they're doing!

This is so important and I'll take pity on those readers who have not got a copy of it on their bookshelf! Here's a one paragraph synopsis of *Making a Difference*:

The emphasis is on improving access and developing practical skills early on in training, with stepping off points at the end of the first year. By autumn 2001, 85% of all nurse-training organisations will be operating the new arrangements. By autumn 2002, it will be standard across the whole of England.

As the NHS Plan calls for similar principles to be applied to education and training for the other health professions and health scientists, you'd better read the rest of it and find out what is going to happen to you!

There will be reforms to the health curricula to give everyone working in the NHS the necessary skills and knowledge to respond effectively to the individual needs of patients.

There will be new joint training across professions in communication skills and in NHS principles and organisation. They will form part of a new core curriculum for all NHS staff education programmes.

It ain't what you say, it's the way that you say it . . .

By 2002, it will be a pre-condition of qualification to deliver patient care in the NHS for an individual to demonstrate competence in communication with patients.

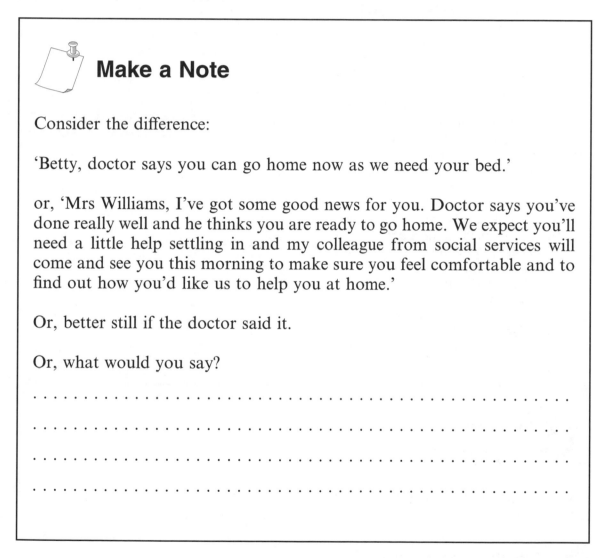

Make a Note

Consider the difference:

'Betty, doctor says you can go home now as we need your bed.'

or, 'Mrs Williams, I've got some good news for you. Doctor says you've done really well and he thinks you are ready to go home. We expect you'll need a little help settling in and my colleague from social services will come and see you this morning to make sure you feel comfortable and to find out how you'd like us to help you at home.'

Or, better still if the doctor said it.

Or, what would you say?

. . . .

. . . .

. . . .

. . . .

A new common foundation programme will be put in place to enable students and staff to switch careers and training paths more easily. Nurses, midwives or therapists who want to become doctors, for example, will no longer have to start their training from scratch.

Here's what the Chief Nursing Officer thinks nursing should be about.

Agree

Disagree

Already doing it

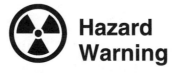

10 key roles for nurses

1   To order diagnostic investigations such as pathology tests and X-rays.
2   To make and receive referrals direct, say, to a therapist or a pain consultant.
3   To admit and discharge patients for specified conditions and within agreed protocols.
4   To manage patient caseloads, say, for diabetes or rheumatology.
5   To run clinics, say, for ophthalmology or dermatology.
6   To prescribe medicines and treatments.
7   To carry out a wide range of resuscitation procedures including defibrillation.
8   To perform minor surgery and outpatient procedures
9   To triage patients, using the latest IT, to the most appropriate health professional.
10   To take a lead in the way local health services are organised and in the way that they are run.

☢️ **Hazard Warning**

Who's gonna do what the nurses used to do?

Can I ask a question?

The NHS Plan says we're all set to have 20 000 more nurses in England but why 20 000 and not 19 000 or 23 000? How did we get to a figure of 20 000?

Has anyone got any ideas?

There are 630 000 nurses on the register. Give or take a few thousand, 300 000 work in the NHS and about 100 000 work outside the NHS. An additional 20 000 nurses is about 6.67% of the current NHS nursing compliment. How did we get to that figure?

> There are 230 000 registered nurses who don't appear to be working. If we could persuade just over 8% of them to come back to the NHS, there would be no problem with the 20 000 target. But it still doesn't explain why 20 000!

We know there are about 15 000 nursing vacancies. Did someone say 'We need 15 000 now, so by the time we reach that number some more will have left or retired, so 20 000 sounds about right!'? We also know that a hugely significant number of nurses are aged over 50 and approaching retirement. Gossip at the RCN says that we need to replace nurses at a rate of about 200 a month but we're only getting 100 trainees into the system.

What about other countries? Comparisons between the UK and other countries are hard to come by. The World Health Organization has some 1998 data but it doesn't include UK figures as we appear not to have supplied them. Strange.

Here's an interpretation of their data with some estimates of our own situation based on a population of 58 million and a working nurse population in the NHS of 300 000.

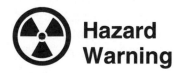 **Hazard Warning**

Beware! This comes with a Lilley health warning! The figures are not European comparisons but have been taken to give a feel for a more global position. Some of the sources are 1993, some are later. You are forgiven for thinking they are not worth a second look, but they might be worth a first look. Taken in the spirit of enquiry and not academia, they are quite interesting.

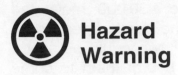

Hazard Warning

Estimates of nurse and midwife numbers per 100 000 head of population – various countries.

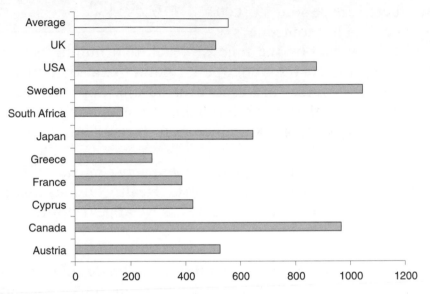

Source: WHO and Economist Digest
Reference point: http://www.who.int/whosis

International comparisons are dangerous and because healthcare systems and methods of funding differ and socio-economic and deprivation statistics vary so much, all comparisons should be taken with a pinch of salt. These data are no different. However, we are still left with the question 'why 20 000 more nurses?'.

Looking across the range of countries it's interesting to speculate what the nurses do in each. In the UK nurses are only just starting to break into the clinical care sector – we have one (or is it two?) nurse surgeons. In the US they are common. We have no (or a couple?) of nurse nephrologists. Europe does.

The whole workforce planning picture becomes very interesting. Will we really be able to hire 20 000 nurses to do what nurses traditionally do and widen their skills into a preserve which has traditionally been the doctor's turf? Does it make more sense to recruit a lower grade of nurse and simply let the doctors get on with it?

A final thought. In the Philippines, from where some UK Trusts have recruited nurses, there are 43 nurses per head of 100 000 population. Sri Lanka has 112.

Leadership

Here's what the NHS Plan says:

'The public consultation provoked a strong call for a "modern matron" figure.'

Turn back the pages to the survey data at the beginning of the book and see what the public actually said. OK, don't bother, here it is again:

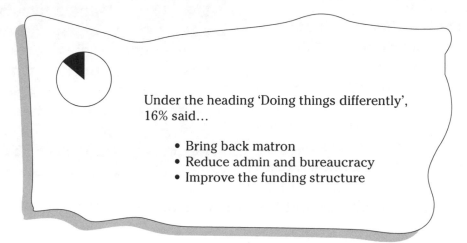

Under the heading 'Doing things differently', 16% said...

- Bring back matron
- Reduce admin and bureaucracy
- Improve the funding structure

Bear in mind that the 16% response includes reducing admin and bureaucracy and improving the funding structure – quite how many people wanted the return of 'matron' is unclear. Perhaps it wasn't a strong call? Incidentally, the staff consultation made no mention of a matron figure whatsoever!

Nevertheless, we are going to get a strong clinical leader with clear authority at ward level. The ward sister or charge nurse will be given authority to resolve clinical issues such as discharge delays, and environmental problems such as poor cleanliness.

By April 2002, every hospital will have senior sisters and charge nurses who are easily identifiable to patients and who will be accountable for a group of wards. They will be in control of the necessary resources to sort out the fundamentals of care, backed up by appropriate administrative support. In the words of the Plan: 'In this way patients' demand for a "modern matron" will be met'.

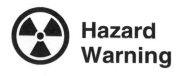 **Hazard Warning**

Evidence-based decision making, eh?

Leaders: how many do you want?

By the way, where are the followers?

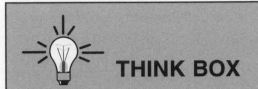

THINK BOX

Is a NHS manager's loyalty to the patient or to political masters? True leaders challenge a system and can make life very uncomfortable for ministers. Remember how ministers reacted when, in 1999, the leaders of the Health Managers' Finance Association challenged funding figures in the NHS?

- By 2004, there will be around 1000 nurse consultants employed in the NHS.
- By then, a first generation of therapist consultants will have started work. They will work with senior hospital doctors, nurses and midwives in drawing up local clinical and referral protocols alongside primary care colleagues.
- The NHS Modernisation Agency will provide management support and training for clinical and medical directors to better equip them for their leadership tasks.
- In place by 2001, a new Leadership Centre for Health operating through the NHS Modernisation Agency, providing tailored support for clinicians and managers with leadership potential.
- Chair and non-executive development care.

Oh, alright, the patients. . .

True or false?

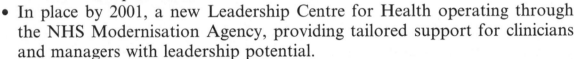

Yup | Maybe | Not where I work

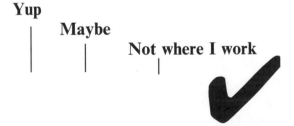

- Patients are the most important people in the health service.
- Patients feel talked at, rather than listened to.
- The NHS is shaped around the convenience and concerns of staff, not patients.

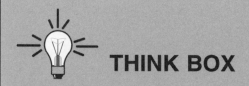

THINK BOX

The NHS Plan wants patients to have more say, know more and participate more in healthcare.

Is this really what the man and woman in the street really wants? There is a dedicated minority, committee creatures and community enthusiasts, who will take the time to become involved. And thank-you to them.

The majority of us want a NHS that is safe, clean, available when we want it and respectful to us when we use it. Somewhere organised that doesn't waste our taxes and somewhere where staff seem happy and genuinely interested in us.

Is this too difficult to deliver without a complex maze of patient and user surveys, focus groups, questionnaires, committees, work groups, case conferences, polls and studies?

What happened to commonsense and peace of mind!

Look out, there's an expert about

Do you know the definition of an 'expert'? Well, '**ex**' is a has-been and a '**(s)pert**' is a drip under pressure . . . beware of experts.

The 'Expert Patient' Programme

- It will require NICE to publish patient-friendly versions of all its clinical guidelines.
- Patients will be helped to navigate the maze of health information through the development of NHS Direct online, digital TV and NHS Direct information points in key public places (includes dentistry).
- More information for patients.
- Greater patient choice.
- Patient advocates and advisers in every hospital.
- Redress over cancelled operations.
- Patient forums and citizen panels in every area.
- New national panel to advise on major reorganisations of hospitals.
- Stronger regulation of professional standards.

- Letters between clinicians about an individual patient's care will be copied to the patient as of right.
- Smart cards for patients, allowing easier access to health records.

Choosing a GP

Yes, yes – patients can do it already . . . but how do they do it? If they move to a new area, how will they find out about the local GPs? If you're a young mum, I guess you'd ask other mums at the school gates. If you're a senior citizen and wanted a GP with a particular interest in the elderly, you might ask at a seniors' club or quiz the neighbours.

To make it easier, GPs will publish new data:

Proposed new data	*Will it make it easier?*
List size	Does this mean a popular doctor has the biggest list, or the doctor with the smallest list can spend more time with each patient?
Accessibility	Public transport, dial-a-ride services, car parking or disabled access? Aren't all surgeries supposed to be in natural communities and have disabled access by law? Oh, what about opening times and weekend surgeries?
Performance against standards in NSFs	Does poor performance mean bad doctoring or that the background health standards in a socially deprived area are bad and therefore case-mix outcome data are skewed?
The number of patients each practice removes from its list	Bad doctoring or $%&&*#! difficult patients?

 Make a Note

What information could GPs publish that will be of real relevance to patients and help them choose a doctor who is interested in them? Consider clinics, specialties, opening times and . . . (over to you!)

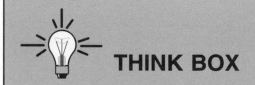

THINK BOX

By 2005, all patients will be able to book every hospital appointment and elective admission, giving them a choice of convenient date and time rather than being assigned a time by the hospital.

What impact will this have on secondary care waiting list and theatre schedule management?

Witch doctor?

Oops, sorry . . . make that 'which doctor?' Hobson's choice.

Prior to 1991, GPs could refer patients to the hospital of their choice. The introduction of the NHS internal market changed that because non-fundholding GPs could no longer automatically refer patients outside their local area – the health authority often made the arrangements.

Since 1999, the creation of PCGs and PCTs means that GPs now collectively decide where to fund services. But does this mean any more choice for the patient? No!

Do patients trust their doctor to make the right choice about the appropriate clinician? Are patients more worried about quality and equity, or locality, travel and the ease of visiting?

Let me remind you. This is from the front of the book and is the data from the national survey comparing what the NHS thinks with what the patients think:

Reduce waiting:

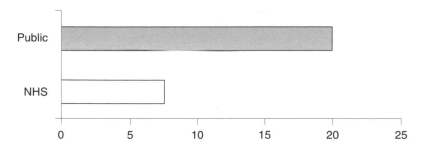

Improve quality:

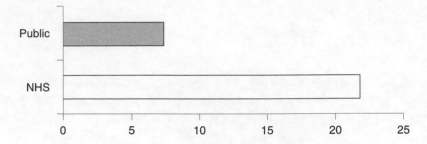

More patient-centred care:

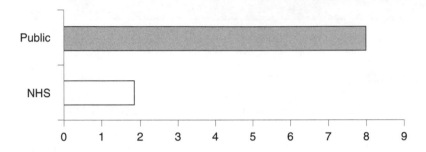

Reduce national variations in care (postcode issues):

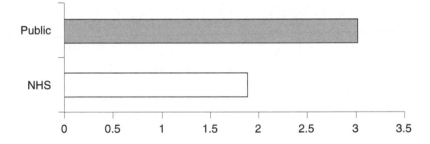

In short, patients want to be treated better, have equal access to treatments, think that NHS quality is fine and that waiting for treatment is a very important factor.

By contrast, NHS staff consider that postcode issues are less important, 'Patient-centred care? Err, what's that?', waiting is only a third of the problem patients think it is and NHS quality is very dodgy.

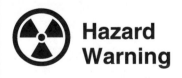 **Hazard Warning**

Another fine example of evidence-based decision making!

SECTION 8

Being in safe hands

The proposals

- A mandatory reporting scheme for adverse healthcare events.
- A single database for analysing and sharing the lessons from incidents and near misses.
- Rapid and robust mechanisms for dealing with under and poor performance among individual doctors.

A National Clinical Assessment Authority will be established as an arms-length Special Health Authority from April 2001. Where concern has arisen locally, it will provide rapid and objective expert assessment of an individual doctor's performance, recommending to the health authority, or employing Trust, educational or other approaches as appropriate.

For the details try a copy of *Supporting Doctors, Protecting Patients*. All doctors employed in, or under contract to, the NHS will, as a condition of contract, be required to participate in annual appraisal and clinical audit from 2001.

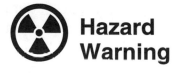 **Hazard Warning**

Will this mean an end to the current arrangement whereby doctors can remain suspended for years while concerns or allegations about their practice are resolved?

Yup!

The NHS Tribunal will be abolished, and the power to suspend or remove GPs from a health authority's list will be devolved to health authorities, subject to a right of appeal to the Family Health Services Appeals Authority.

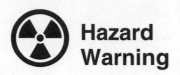 **Hazard Warning**

Beware (if you are a doc) that a consultant's right to appeal against disciplinary action direct to the Secretary of State under the 'paragraph 190' arrangements will end, so that responsibility is devolved from the Secretary of State to NHS Trusts locally, from 2001.

Reforming the General Medical Council – at last

The beleaguered GMC is fighting for survival. Will it still be around in five years?

The GMC seems to be in a state of terminal indecision about what it should be doing and, as such, it has issued a discussion document. Interestingly they have invited comment and answers not to the whole of the document, but on specific questions.

> Most polling gurus will tell you, privately, that they've done it this way so they can shape the answers the way they want them.

The GMC proposes that doctors have a 'folder' into which are inserted qualifications, postgraduate learning and a Boys Scout badge collection of other memorabilia. (Why am I so cynical whenever the GMC surfaces?)

It's proposed that the folders are reviewed every five years. Five years!! Time enough for a Shipman-wanna-be to do in another 15 patients, a geriatric pathologist to get another 2000 tests wrong and a gynaecologist to slash his way through another 20 women.

Reviewed by whom? You may well ask! Two doctors and a lay person – now, there's a surprise. The docs outnumber the customers once again! When will the GMC learn that the old boy's club days are over.

It's not only me who gets excited about the GMC – even the BMA membership has passed a 'no confidence' motion in the GMC, not once but twice! If you consider that a primary aim of the GMC is to protect doctors, what does this tell you about how the GMC is regarded? Why doesn't government just nail up the front door and let a patient branch of the Commission for Health Improvement take over?

Anyway, here are the questions. There's room for your comments but I couldn't resist adding a few of my own – just in case you couldn't tell where I was coming from!

Question	Here's what I say	What do you say?
Do you agree with the principles of revalidation?	Yup	
Do you agree with the contents of the folder?	Neutral, it's little more than the sort of personnel file you'd find anywhere in industry, as long as it's open to the public to inspect	
Should anonymous complaints be included in the folder?	Yes, as they might establish a trend	
. . . the principles underpinning the link between appraisal and regular review . . .	Sure	
Should GPs be revalidated every five years?	No, every year just like airline pilots. . . and include a medical please	
. . . the revalidation group recording required actions on the revalidation certificate submitted to the GMC . . .	Yup, and available to the public	
What would be the appropriate lay involvement on the revalidation group?	Lay dominated with technical advice as required	
Arrangements for the regular review and five year recommendations for locums?	No, locums are often dangerous and frequently exposed to out-of-hours problems requiring a higher standard of doctoring	
Arrangements for revalidation of doctors who do not need the exercise registration in order to perform their job?	Then don't call them a doctor, find another title	
Arrangements for retired doctors?	A glass of gin and a gold watch. Thanks and bye bye	

Question	Here's what I say	What do you say?
Arrangements for doctors working abroad?	Same as working at home – use the Internet to do the job	
How to distinguish on the register between doctors who are participating in revalidation and those who are not?	No participation, no mention on the register	
The privileges of registration that might be retained by doctors who are not participating in revalidation?	None	
Arrangements for returning to practice?	Re-exam, medical – the works	
Inclusion of revalidation date on the register?	Yup	
Time limitations on the disclosure of past GMC findings?	None	
Discretionary powers for the committee investigating a doctor's participation in revalidation to award costs for or against the doctor?	Yup	

The GMC should also explore the introduction of a civil burden of proof and make other reforms if it's to genuinely protect patients. Government and Parliament will have to judge whether the GMC's proposed reforms, following its own consultation process, will protect patients and restore public and professional confidence.

So, write to your MP and tell him what you think . . .

UK Council of Health Regulators

A UK Council of Health Regulators will be established which will include the:

- GMC (as mentioned in the NHS Plan – the very fact that the GMC is written about in these terms leads me to believe the GMC is safe, whatever happens. Will the government have the guts to take on the GMC, a bastion of the medical establishment?)
- successor bodies to the UKCC for Nursing, Midwifery and Health Visiting
- Council for Professions Supplementary to Medicine
- General Dental Council

- General Optical Council
- Royal Pharmaceutical Society
- General Osteopaths Council
- General Chiropractic Council

. . . and patients. Oh yes, I nearly forgot, we were talking about patients . . .

Patient Advocacy and Liaison Service (PALS)

A Patient Advocacy and Liaison Service (PALS) will be established in every Trust, beginning with every major hospital. PALS will have an annual national budget of around £10 million.

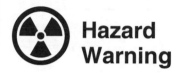 **Hazard Warning**

Bad idea! PALS will be Trust apparatchiks.

Situated in the main reception area of hospitals the new patient advocate team will be a clearly identifiable information point and a welcoming point for patients and carers. Patient advocates will act as independent facilitators handling patient and family concerns, have direct access to the chief executive and the powers to negotiate immediate solutions.

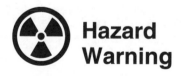 **Hazard Warning**

These new arrangements are at the expense of the Community Health Councils. Now while it's true that some CHCs were often politically driven and ineffective, more interested in politics than patients, many did a good job and, most significantly, they were genuinely independent. PALS will be on the pay roll and open to manipulation – hence they'll have to be really tough in withstanding pressure from within the Trust.

In mental health and learning disability services, the PALS team will build on and support current specialist advocacy services.

What can a PAL do?

- It will steer patients and families towards the complaints process where necessary.
- It will take on the roles which CHCs currently fulfil in supporting complainants.
- It will work with other organisations, such as Citizens Advice Bureaux.

What's in it for patients?

- The right to redress when things go wrong.
- From 2002, if a patient's operation is cancelled by the hospital on the day of surgery for non-clinical reasons, the hospital will have to offer another binding date within a maximum of the next 28 days or fund the patient's treatment at the time and hospital of the patient's choice.

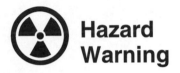

Hazard Warning

What about notes, tests and liaison? Look out Harley Street, do you have enough beds!

- A new complaints procedure – let's just hope it's better than the last one.

Complaints

Make a Note

What are your experiences of the existing complaints procedure? How can it be improved and made less adversarial and more transparent? What part does the 'blame culture' play? Should we look at a no fault system like they have in New Zealand? Critics say it's expensive but should that be the key determinant when patient complaints are being considered? Should patients and their relatives and carers have to trail around the courts for years?

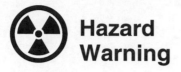

Hazard Warning

Complaints cost but claims cost more . . .

In 1996, the National Audit Office estimated the cost of clinical negligence at £220 million a year. The mutual insurance scheme for Trusts (called the Clinical Negligence Scheme) reported that it had 634 open claims on its books, with an estimated value of £180 million. So it's next to broke, isn't it!

What do complainants want?

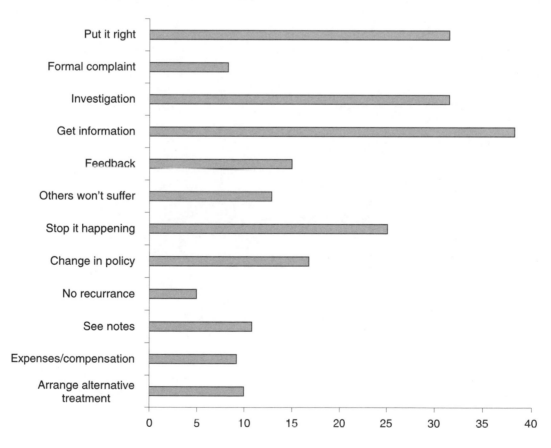

This is an extract from some fascinating work by Sally Lloyd-Bostock (Reader in Law at the University of Birmingham), who conducted an analysis of complaints letters.

In many cases she found that the complainant had no idea what they wanted the Trust to do, or what they hoped to achieve by complaining. (Good luck PALS!)

This is only a small part of some very interesting work and you can find the rest in a book called *Medical Mishaps* (Open University Press). There's a little stocking filler for Christmas!

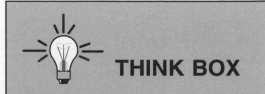

THINK BOX

A hospital consultant once said 'Clinical complaints, about clinicians, must be dealt with by clinicians. What do managers know about treating patients?' It's a bit like policemen insisting only the police can investigate the police. Agree or disagree?

Consultants *vs* GPs – what do we complain about?

More stuff from that book again, this time by contributors Judith Allsop and Linda Mulcahy:

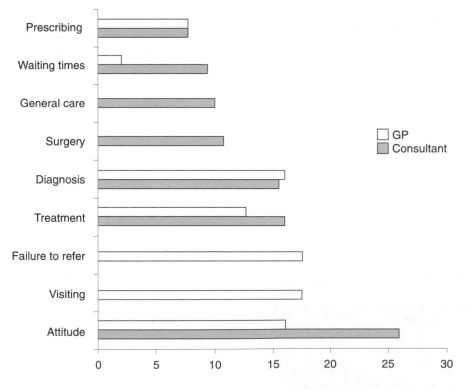

Source: *Medical Mishaps* (Open University Press)

Looks like they're as bad as each other!

What is the impact of a complaint on a doctor? Here are some quotes from that book again:

'I had sleepless nights – I was devastated. Colleagues told me not to worry, but my reputation was being questioned.'

'Complaints are very hurtful. One gets emotionally involved because they strike at one's perception of oneself as a doctor.'

'The greatest sense is futility – why bother to try when resources are inadequate and patients are complaining?'

Here's another very interesting insight into complaints (again taken from that terrific book on the subject) that gives us a feel of how weak the existing complaints procedure is and indicating what we might do to resolve the problem:

'The consultant study showed that where they were able to conceal receipt of a complaint from a manager, they often did so. In theory managers should be informed of all formal complaints within a hospital, but in 60% of the complaints addressed to the responsible consultant, the doctor dealt with the complaint without contacting a manager. One of the main reasons consultants gave for not referring complaints to managers was that they did not believe that managers had "the right" to handle clinical complaints. In other words they acted to protect their individual and group autonomy.'

Closing ranks? Now you can see why complaints statistics make no sense and consultant–manager relationships are so poor.

How would you feel if someone complains about you?

Yup!

- Frightened? – about your job, your reputation, where the complaint will go
- Injured? – the complainant doesn't understand the grief they've caused
- Irritated? – especially if the complaint is unjustified or involves something trivial

When do you get around to the most important bit – admitting that you might just be wrong? Just remember that doctors are no different from the rest of us.

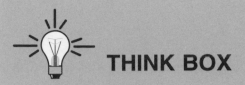

THINK BOX

What have we learned? Perhaps that any new system has to be fast and focused for patients and fair to doctors, and that the basis of a complaint must change from being a threat to competency to being a contribution to doing things better.

A new NHS Charter

By 2001, a new NHS Charter (replacing the current Patients' Charter) will make it clear how people can access NHS services, set out the NHS commitment to patients and define the rights and responsibilities of patients within the NHS.

As it stands now, the only right a patient has is to be registered with a GP. However, that is set to change.

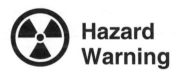

Hazard Warning

From 2 October 2000, an NHS body in England and Wales that acts incompatibly, in any way, with the rights set out in the European Convention on Human Rights, will be acting unlawfully.

Human Rights Act, Section 6

What are the rights?

	Area covered	Some likely impacts
Article 2	. . . the right to life	Do not resuscitate policies
Article 3	. . . not to be subjected to inhuman or degrading treatment or punishment	Mental health policy
Article 5	. . . the right to liberty and the security of the person	Mental health policy
Article 6	. . . the right to a fair and public hearing	Staff disputes
Article 8	. . . the right to respect for family and private life, home and correspondence	Email traffic at work
Article 9	. . . the right to freedom of thought, conscience and religion	HR strategies
Article 10	. . . the right to freedom of expression	HR strategies, confidentiality and whistle blowing
Article 11	. . . the right to freedom of peaceful assembly and to join a trade union	HR and transfer of undertakings for PFI staff
Article 12	. . . the right to marry and found a family	IVF treatment
Article 14	. . . the right not to be discriminated against on the grounds of, and in relation to, the enjoyment of conventional rights	Children's services, access to all drugs no matter how costly, NICE and all the rest!

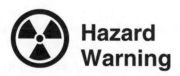 **Hazard Warning**

The impact of the Human Rights Act is too complicated to go into here. However, there's an excellent workbook, shortly to be published by Radcliffe Medical Press, written by someone I'm too modest to name. Seriously though, it's a complicated issue and has the potential to overturn some well-established thinking in the NHS. Blanket policies on care access are probably in trouble. In short, don't get left out or caught out by the human rights stuff!

Consent

Following criticism that patients may not be properly involved in decisions about resuscitation, every hospital will have to have a local resuscitation policy based on guidelines published by the BMA and Royal College of Nursing.

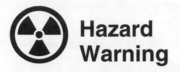

Hazard Warning

These guidelines are disputed by a number of doctor groups and, perhaps, cannot be taken to represent the view of the whole profession. There's an alliance of doctors who do not agree with them – check with your doctors on where they stand.

And finally

- All NHS Trusts, PCGs and PCTs will have to ask patients and carers for their views on the services they have received.
- All patients leaving hospital will be given the opportunity to record their views about the standards of care they have received, in writing or electronically through new bedside TV information services.
- Every local NHS organisation, as well as care homes, will be required to publish, in a new Patient Prospectus, an annual account of the views received from patients – and the actions taken as a result.

The Patient Prospectus will set out:

- the range of local services available and the ratings they have received from patients
- and the place they occupy under the Performance Assessment Framework.

Also:

- a Patients' Forum will be established in every NHS Trust and PCT to provide direct input from patients into how local NHS services are run
- patients will have direct representation on every NHS Trust Board – elected by the Patients' Forum
- the Patients' Forum will have half of its members drawn from local patient groups and voluntary organisations
- the other half will be randomly drawn from respondents to the Trust's annual patient survey
- the Forum will be supported by the new Patient Advocate and Liaison

Service, and will have the right to visit and inspect any aspect of the Trust's care at any time
- PALS staff and Forum members will have access to the new NHS Leadership Centre's programmes.

The democratic deficit – spot the difference

Local government spends millions of pounds of public money on vital services and is overseen by members who are elected by the community to run affairs on their behalf.

The NHS spends millions of pounds of public money on vital services and is overseen by members who are not elected by the community to run affairs on their behalf.

So:

- chief executives of NHS organisations will be required to attend the main local authority all-party scrutiny committee at least twice annually if requested
- the power to refer major planned changes in local NHS services to the Secretary of State will transfer from CHCs to the all-party scrutiny committees of elected local authorities. The council scrutiny committees – which must meet in public – will be able to refer contested major service reconfigurations to the new Independent Reconfiguration Panel.

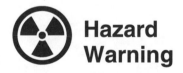 **Hazard Warning**

These are big changes which could make it very difficult to reconfigure services. Get to know the local council and don't just meet with them twice a year – make regular liaison routine and make sure they understand the day-to-day issues that go into making up the big picture. The local council is no longer 'that lot down the road'.

The Committee on the English Regions last met in 1978. In 1998, the Tories floated the idea of balancing the government's package of devolution reforms by turning Westminster into an English Parliament. William Hague has since dropped the idea. However, the Lib Dems seem keen and Whitehall gossips talk of regional assemblies being in the next Labour manifesto. So, are regional assemblies far off?

The government feels that patients and (as they are wont to call us) citizens, have had too little influence at every level of the NHS. As a result of this Plan, each health authority area will be required to establish an independent local advisory forum chosen from area residents, to provide a sounding board for determining health priorities and policies, including the Health Improvement Programme.

SECTION 9

Working with the private sector

The headline in Issue 13 (Summer 2000) of the Independent Healthcare Association's magazine said it all:

IHA in biggest coup of the century

Thursday, 15th June was a momentous day for independent health and social care.

On that day, the Secretary of State for Health, Alan Milburn, gave a radio interview which signalled a landmark in the delivery of health and social care in the UK.

It marked the end of a long, backstage struggle by this association to put the sector firmly on the political map. But it also heralded the beginning of a new era of joint working with both the NHS and local government.

Appearing on the *Today* programme Mr Milburn spoke of a 'concordat' between government and representatives of the independent health and social care sector.

A big coup and a big crow . . . unlikely to go down well with those parts of the Labour Party who still regard the private sector as the enemy.

The NHS already spends over £1 billion each year on buying care and specialist services from hospitals, nursing homes and hospices run by private companies and charities.

So, what's in this 'concordat' then?

- A set of national guidelines to help PCGs and PCTs when they commission services.
- **Elective care**: this could take the form of NHS doctors and nurses using the operating theatres and facilities in private hospitals, or it could mean the NHS buying in certain services.
- **Critical care**: this will allow the NHS and private sector to transfer patients to and from each other whenever clinically appropriate.
- **Intermediate care**: this will involve the private and voluntary sector developing and making available facilities to support the government's strategy for better preventive and rehabilitation services.

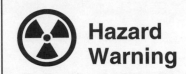

Hazard Warning

Don't the same docs and often the same nurses work in the NHS and the private sector? Won't this act as an incentive to build up NHS waiting lists and make a nice few quid for the local private hospital?

Make a Note

Clear cost arrangements, particularly when patients are transferred as emergency cases, will need to be established before the concordat takes effect locally.

Do you have sufficiently robust accounting systems to be able to compare and contract with the private sector?

R&D

Advances in science and technology have revolutionised modern medicine, providing the antibiotics, vaccines, modern anaesthetics and pharmaceuticals that have helped transform our lives.

The manufacturers of these advances make millions out of the NHS, so does the NHS have a responsibility to contribute? The Plan thinks it does:

- by developing a strong set of national research and development programmes
- a collaborative role in realising the benefits of genetics
- through a long-term study of the interactions of genetics and the environment in common adult diseases such as cancer, heart disease and diabetes
- through the Human Genetics Commission, advising on the social, ethical and legal implications of developments in genetics and engaging the public in considering these questions
- commissioning NHS R&D in new centres of excellence to evaluate all aspects of the emerging developments in genetics, from laboratory testing to the requirement for counselling of patients.

The Confederation of British Industry estimates that temporary sickness costs business over £10 billion annually and the burden is carried by employers and the NHS. Back pain accounts for 119 million days of certified incapacity and also consumes 12 million GP consultations and 800 000 inpatient days of hospital care.

A new set of services, NHSplus, will be developed as part of the NHS Plan. A portfolio of NHS occupational health services will be identified and then be bought, in whole or in part, by employers to improve the health of their employees.

NHSplus will be established as a national agency and the business plan will ensure that these new services are provided at no cost to the taxpayer, building on local services provided by hospitals and PCTs. Surpluses will be reinvested in the expansion and improvement of NHS services.

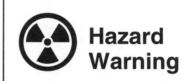 **Hazard Warning**

Oh, no! Whenever the NHS goes into business it loses a fortune. Tell me it won't be like that this time!

 Make a Note

Could you sell occupational health services to the firms in your area? Consider drawing up a business plan which is cost neutral to the NHS and will make a profit. Yes, I know the Plan uses the word 'surplus' but a surplus isn't a profit – see, they're in a mess already! Can you save them?

SECTION 10

Waiting around

Waiting for treatment, waiting to see a GP, waiting to be seen in a casualty department, waiting to get into hospital and, sometimes, waiting to get out of hospital – top of the list for patients. But it's not a view shared by NHS staff – remember the NHS survey?

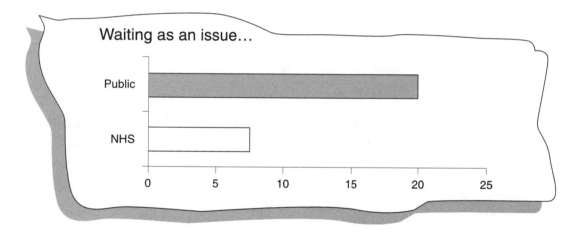

Waiting as an issue...

By the end of 2000, NHS Direct, the 24-hour telephone helpline, will have gone nationwide. The idea? Get more people to sort themselves out. By 2004, NHS Direct will be providing health information via digital TV as well as the telephone and Internet. By then, there will be over 500 NHS Direct information points providing touchscreen information and advice about health and the health service, in places like shopping centres and railway stations.

Docs seem to moan end-lessly about NHS Direct, but it has a 98% approval rating with the public!

Starting in 2001, patients will get greater access to authoritative information about how they can care for themselves and their families under the aegis of NHSplus, which will produce and kite-mark books, leaflets and other written material.

By 2001, there will be new quality standards and closer integration too between NHS Direct and GP out-of-hours services. By 2004, a single phone call to NHS Direct will be a one-stop gateway to out-of-hours healthcare, with the passing on of calls, where necessary, to the appropriate GP co-operative or deputising service.

By 2002, all NHS Direct sites will refer people, where appropriate, to help from their local pharmacy. There will be better out-of-hours pharmacy services and:

> A week after the NHS Plan was published, NHS waiting list statistics were published – and they were up again. Apparently, seven hospitals are responsible for 23% of the waiting list over-run. I know each of the hospitals and staff who work in each of them and they are diligent, good people.
>
> Lord Hunt of King's Health, Lords' Minister for Health and once CEO of NAHAT (the forerunner of the NHS Confederation), has ordered in a CHI hit squad to sort them out. I wonder how they feel. I bet they look forward to going to work on Monday mornings.

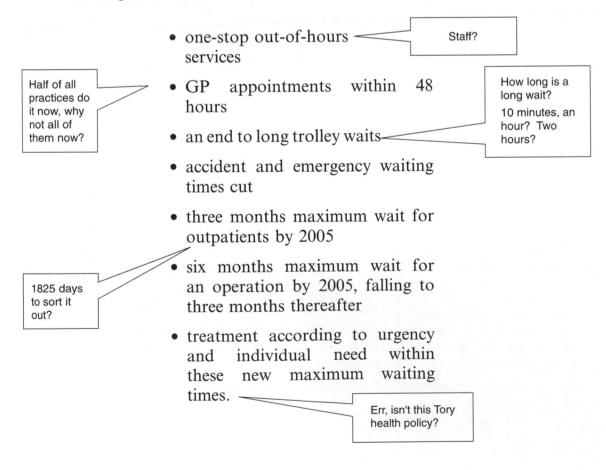

- one-stop out-of-hours services
- GP appointments within 48 hours
- an end to long trolley waits
- accident and emergency waiting times cut
- three months maximum wait for outpatients by 2005
- six months maximum wait for an operation by 2005, falling to three months thereafter
- treatment according to urgency and individual need within these new maximum waiting times.

Staff?

Half of all practices do it now, why not all of them now?

How long is a long wait?
10 minutes, an hour? Two hours?

1825 days to sort it out?

Err, isn't this Tory health policy?

Meanwhile, down at the pharmacy:

• availability of a wider range of over-the-counter medicines

• by 2004, every PCG and PCT will have schemes in place so that people get more help from pharmacists in using their medicines. Nationwide repeat dispensing schemes so that obtaining repeat prescriptions is easier for patients with chronic conditions.

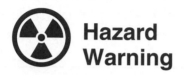 **Hazard Warning**

'By 2004, consultants who previously worked only in hospitals will be delivering approximately 4 million outpatient consultations in primary care and community settings.'

Easy to say, not easy to do. What about the kit and bits and pieces they need for examinations and diagnosis? Health records, test results, bookings, admissions – all need to be sorted before this can happen. Only robust IT systems can enable the peripatetic consultant. And, by the way, what about training juniors? Does this mean one doctor and a trainee riding shotgun?

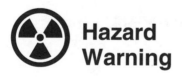 **Hazard Warning**

'Up to 1000 specialist GPs will be taking referrals from fellow GPs for conditions in specialties such as ophthalmology, orthopaedics, dermatology and ear, nose and throat surgery. They will also be able to undertake diagnostic procedures such as endoscopy.'

All the evidence suggests that the more you do, the better you get – that's why we have specialists! The thought of gung-ho GPs having a go at this and that, doing a few bits and pieces every month fills me with dread. Is this about making the life of a bored GP more fun or is it about delivering safe treatments to patients?

And, anyway, whilst the GPs are away being specialists, who is going to do what the GP used to do?

Dentistry

Dentists are as rare as hen's teeth in some parts of the country but nothing is left out of the NHS Plan!

'The government is firmly committed to making high-quality NHS dentistry available to all who want it by September 2001. The initiatives we have taken since 1997 have already made a real difference but more needs to be done. In future, NHS Direct will help direct patients to NHS dentistry. The government will fund more dental access centres and improvements to dental practices. It will reward dentists' commitment to the NHS and foster better quality services for patients, making NHS dentistry a modern and truly national service again.'

 Make a Note

Health authorities will take the lead in delivering the changes which patients expect. So sayeth the Plan. Can you make an estimate of unmet demand for dentistry? Has fluoridation and diet made dentistry less of an issue than it was?

If you think dentistry isn't as important as it was, take a look at this:

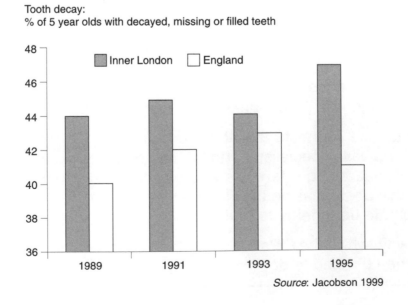

Tooth decay:
% of 5 year olds with decayed, missing or filled teeth

Source: Jacobson 1999

Who invented the phrase 'bed blocker'?

Isn't it tough enough to be elderly, unwell, unsure, worried about the future and on top of all that, insulted with the phrase 'bed blocker'. Work hard all your life, pay hundreds of thousands of pounds in taxes and when you need some treatment and a bit of TLC, all you get is membership of the bed blocker club.

Well the Plan says it's going to end widespread bed blocking (by 2004) and, hopefully, put an end to the use of the dreadful phrase.

How are they going to do it? With a discharge plan! Don't we have them now?

Make a Note

What's the situation with discharge plans where you work?

- Does it include an assessment of care needs?
- Is it developed from the beginning of the patient's hospital admission?
- Do patients wait for assessment, support at home, adaptations, equipment or package of care?

If you are not doing all that now (and why not) you'd better figure out a way to do it because that will become the new norm.

Off your trolley

By 2004, no-one should be waiting more than four hours in A&E from arrival to admission, transfer or discharge. At least, that's the plan. If it works, average waiting times in A&E will fall to 75 minutes.

And here's how! It will involve major changes to the way that hospitals work, including:

- more staff
- the creation of medical assessment and admissions units in all hospitals

- new working practices
- nurses taking on new roles including the right to admit patients and order diagnostic procedures
- patients with minor injuries treated by appropriately trained primary care staff working in A&E.

Make a Note

In the US, where in some inner cities they've given up on any semblance of primary care, there is a new grade of worker in the A&E department – 'hospitalists', part nurse, part technician and part doctor.

Consider how that grade of worker might solve some UK problems.

Beating the clock and the calendar

Did you know, at present, the average wait to see a consultant for an outpatient appointment is seven weeks and that the average time people wait for an operation is three months?

The ones that wait much longer attract the headlines. Some wait much longer – up to 18 months for inpatient treatment.

So, why are we waiting? There are several reasons for long waiting times:

- resources
- equipment
- staff to carry out enough treatments and operations
- some conditions have particular problems.

For example, four specialties account for most of the long waits: orthopaedics; dermatology; ear, nose and throat problems; and eye conditions.

On a national level, waiting lists for the NHS are a way of balancing supply and demand, of matching the volume of care it can provide to the number of people wanting treatment. And at a local level, waiting lists have ensured that consultants always have a flow of patients to treat.

Tests, results and diagnosis are not matched up to provide a complete and integrated service and the scheduling of clinics and theatre lists has been wasteful.

Make a Note

The introduction of on-the-spot booking systems will not just make getting a hospital appointment more convenient for patients. It will also act as a driver for much more fundamental reform.

Booking appointments force hospitals to organise their clinic slots and theatre sessions differently. The question is, will it be more productive? Is it more productive to have a patient-driven list, or a list driven by assembling similar procedures in groups?

What's the likely impact on patient-driven booking systems where you work?

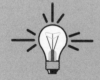

THINK BOX

One of the big reasons for loss of productivity, particularly in outpatients, is the DNS – 'did not show'. Patients who ignore appointments and fail to cancel or turn up. Should that behaviour (without good reason) go unpenalised? What sort of penalty could you introduce?

- Put such patients at the back of the queue?
- Charge for the next appointment?
- Name and shame patients on a list in reception or in local hospitals?
- Your ideas
- . . .
- . . .
- None of the above!

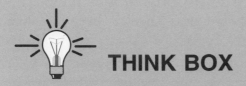

THINK BOX

By the end of 2005, waiting lists for hospital appointments and admission will be abolished and replaced with booking systems giving all patients a choice of convenient time, within a guaranteed maximum waiting time.

Isn't this simply a smart way of doing away with the political embarrassment of waiting lists, targets and press pressure?

As a first step towards this, all hospitals will, by April 2001, have booking systems in place covering two procedures within their major specialties. Assuming that GP referrals remain broadly in line with the current trend in the growth of referrals, then the maximum waiting time for a routine outpatient appointment will be halved from over six months now, to three months.

Urgent cases will continue to be treated much faster in accordance with clinical need. This could mean that the average time for an outpatient appointment falls to five weeks and the maximum wait for inpatient treatment will be cut from 18 months now, to six months.

Make a Note

The eventual objective, by 2008, is to reduce the maximum wait for any stage of treatment to three months.

What additional resources are you likely to need to meet this objective where you work? Too big a question? Try breaking it down specialty by specialty.

If we're having trouble meeting demand, how about stopping folk getting ill in the first place?

Seems like a good idea . . . can there be a greater injustice than the life expectancy of a boy born into the bottom social class to be over nine years less than a boy born into the most affluent social class?

Take a look at this:

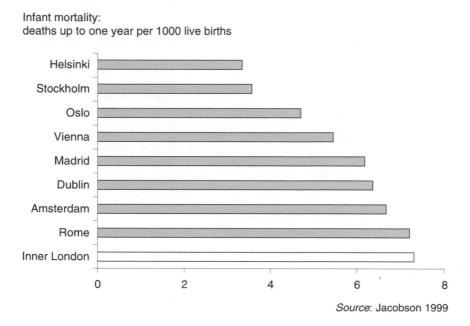

Infant mortality:
deaths up to one year per 1000 live births

Source: Jacobson 1999

Good health at the very beginning of life is the foundation for health throughout life. It's now recognised that women's health in infancy can affect the health of their children. Although infant mortality rates have improved over recent years, the English rate remains above the European average. Infant mortality rates vary widely across health authorities in England, with the highest health authority rate being three and a half times that of the lowest rate. There are also large variations in infant mortality rates by social class of father and ethnic origin of mother. Infants born to fathers in unskilled or semi-skilled occupations have a mortality rate 1.6 times higher than those in professional or managerial occupations. Children of women born in Pakistan are twice as likely to die in their first year than children of women born in the UK.

The worst health problems in our country will not be tackled without first dealing with their fundamental causes. This means tackling disadvantage in all its forms – poverty, lack of educational attainment, unemployment, discrimination and social exclusion.

It means recognising the specific health needs of different groups, including people with disabilities and minority ethnic groups. In fact, a whole new approach.

The NHS is a sickness service buts needs to become a wellness service – encouraging and persuading people that being healthy is more fun than being sick is a job the NHS has never done.

Estimates put the cost to the NHS of poor diet, lack of exercise and smoking at 30% of the treatment budget. Is it too much to ask folk to take some exercise, eat sensibly and stop smoking?

If this is an issue that interests you, then you must make a point of adding the White Paper, *Saving Lives: Our Healthier Nation,* to your reading list.

To tackle some of these issues is beyond local health planners. We spend £1.7 billion a year on the effects of obesity and £1.5 billion a year on smoking-related diseases. Costs are going up all the time.

New drugs for obesity and smoking cessation could bust the pharmacy budget.

In his last budget, and for the first time, the Chancellor introduced the concept of hypothecation into the health funding equation. He put up the price of cigarette duty and passed it on to the NHS.

A mixed blessing? It gives permission to smokers to carry on coughing: 'I'm doing my bit for the NHS'.

The treasury takes £10 billion a year from cigarette smokers – half the defence budget.

No wonder they won't do the real things that need to be done to stop us lighting up.

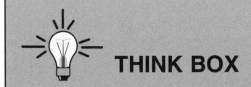

THINK BOX

Is smoking or obesity a lifestyle issue? Do they do such damage to people that investing in a few high-price drugs to help them now, might save us a lot of treatment costs later on?

Seven in 10 smokers want to give up, but smoking still kills 120 000 people a year. It's the leading single cause of avoidable ill health and early death and the biggest single cause of the difference in death rates between rich and poor. Smoking in pregnancy reduces birthweight and contributes to peri-natal mortality.

About time too!

By 2001, for the first time, the NHS will provide a comprehensive smoking cessation service. Nicotine replacement therapy (NRT) will be available on prescription from GPs to complement the newly available smoking cessation treatment, buproprion (Zyban). NICE will be asked to advise GPs on the most appropriate and cost-effective prescribing regimes for nicotine replacement therapy and buproprion, including duration and targeting.

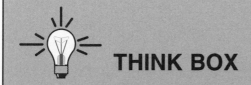

THINK BOX

If you can afford to smoke, can't you afford to give up? Should the NHS pay for smoking cessation treatments?

The Committee on the Safety of Medicines will be asked to consider whether NRT can be made available for general sale rather than only through pharmacies or on prescription.

Specialist smoking cessation services will focus on heavily dependent smokers needing intensive support, and on pregnant female smokers as part of ante-natal care.

For the first time ever, local targets will now be reinforced by the creation of national health inequalities targets designed to narrow the health gap in childhood and throughout life between socio-economic groups.

An apple for teacher

No an apple for the pupil. Every child between four and six will be given a piece of fresh fruit every day at school. Are you old enough to remember free school milk? I am. I also remember the name of the minister who decided it was no longer necessary – Margaret Thatcher.

To underpin the national work on cutting inequalities, by 2002 a new health poverty index will be developed that combines data about health status, access to health services, uptake of preventive services and the opportunities to pursue and maintain good health, such as access to affordable nutritious food, physical activity and a safe, clean environment.

In health there is the inverse care law where communities in greatest need are least likely to receive the health services that they require. This still applies in many parts of the country.

Inequity in access to services is not restricted to social class and geography – people in minority ethnic communities are less likely to receive the services they need. Many deprived communities are less likely to receive heart surgery, hip replacements and screening services than affluent ones.

At the heart of the problem lies the weighted capitation formula used to distribute NHS funding. By 2003, it will be reviewed to include these issues and a new way of distributing resources to address inequities in primary care services should be in place.

Make a Note

There are 50% more GPs in Kingston, Richmond or Oxfordshire than there are in Barnsley or Sunderland after adjusting for the age and needs of their respective populations.

What are the reasons? Is it about middle class, well-educated, white doctors not wanting to set up shop in downtown or run down areas? Is the answer to recruit more doctors from different social classes, age groups and ethnic backgrounds?

How are GPs distributed in your area? What are the factors that mitigate against expansion of primary care in some areas?

The new Medical Education Standards Board will track the number and distribution of doctors in primary care. The Medical Practices Committee will be abolished and replaced with a single resource allocation formula covering all NHS spending, including general medical services non-cash limited expenditure.

To improve the equitable distribution of GPs and primary care staff, 200 new Personal Medical Services (PMS) schemes will be created principally in disadvantaged communities by 2004. New incentives will be developed to help recruit and retain good staff in disadvantaged areas.

Make a Note

What are the incentives likely to bring about this change? Is it just about money? What are the other factors?

Through the NHS Performance Assessment Framework the NHS will address local inequalities, including issues such as access to services for black and ethnic minority communities.

By 2003, a free and nationally available translation and interpretation service will be available in all NHS premises through NHS Direct.

Make a Note

What are the equality and access issues in your area? Think about all the issues, not just language. A single mother with no telephone, two young children, marooned in a tower block in an area with poor public transport may have just as much trouble accessing the surgery as an elderly person. Religion often creates a barrier, for example, for women who must be accompanied when out of doors.

We are what we eat

Poor nutrition leads to low birthweight and poor weight gain in the first year of life, which in turn contributes to the later development of disease, particularly heart disease.

Increased fruit and vegetable consumption is considered the second most effective strategy (behind giving up smoking) in reducing the risk of cancer, and it has major preventive benefits for heart disease too.

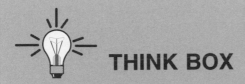

THINK BOX

Do you eat at least five portions of fruit and vegetables a day? It could lead to estimated reductions of up to 20% in overall deaths from chronic disease. In the UK, average consumption is about three portions a day, and a fifth of children eat no fruit at all in a week.

What about all those pre-prepared meals and junk food? Look out for initiatives aimed at the food industry (including manufacturers and caterers), designed to improve the overall balance of diet and reduce the amounts of salt, fat and sugar in processed foods.

Drugs, alcohol abuse and related crime

Perhaps the biggest curse of them all:

- there are up to 200 000 problem drug misusers in the UK
- no more than half are in contact with treatment services

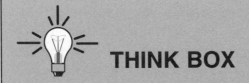

THINK BOX

There are a host of targets and initiatives in the Plan but surely the real issue, particularly in relation to drugs, is how are we going to deal with the problem in the future?

The Drugs Tsar looks no nearer to solving the problem as drug dealers move uptown following the money in wealthy communities. Recent reports estimate that a third of children have been offered hard drugs.

Is this a police, health or legal issue?

What's the best outcome we can expect? All the drug dealers in jail and drugs banished from society? Or the decriminalisation of drugs and a government imposed drugs tax? Which is most likely or can you envisage another scenario?

- there are up to 2300 drug-related deaths a year
- the figure has been rising since 1980.

The government is committed to:

- reducing the proportion of people under the age of 25 using class A drugs by 25% by 2005 and 50% by 2008
- increasing the number of problem drug misusers in treatment by 66% by 2005 and 100% by 2008
- targeting education and prevention activities, intervening before people develop the habits which do so much damage
- strengthening treatment services for drug misusers by setting up a new National Treatment Agency which is accountable to the Department of Health
- pooling the resources spent on drug misuser services by health and other agencies.

Somehow I still have a sense of gloom about drugs.

However, I'll try and cheer myself up by thinking about the Healthy Communities Collaborative which is designed to spread best practice under the aegis of the new Modernisation Agency, using evidence from the Health Development Agency and the successful formula already in place in the Cancer Collaborative and the Primary Care Collaborative.

SECTION 11

Cancer

Why is cancer still at the top of the list? For years men and women have sold cakes, run marathons and children have donated their pocket money towards research to beat cancer. Why do we appear no further forward?

Cancer kills 100 000 people a year and unskilled workers are twice as likely to die from the disease as professionals.

We have some of the worst survival rates for cancer

But do we? Here are a few snippets from what one of our leading public health doctors, Dr Harry Burns (Director of Public Health, Greater Glasgow Health Board), told the NHS Confederation Conference in June 2000:

- It's impossible to say, on the basis of the published data, how cancer mortality varies between European countries.
- The Eurocare Study II, used as the basis for comparison, does not compare like with like.
- Some European data are so poor, it's not considered good enough for inclusion in the study.
- French data show only data for survival from areas where data are good enough and from those willing to be included.
- France only includes the Departments of Côte d'Or, Doubs, Isère and Somme – just 3% of the population.
- In Germany only one cancer registry made it into Eurocare – the Saarland registry which covers 1.7% of the population.
- Swiss figures only cover Basle and Geneva – 12% of the population.
- Only Scotland and Denmark use the same method of recording and, interestingly, have similar mortality rates.

- Only 49% of the English population is included – East Anglia, Mersey, Oxford, South Thames, Wessex, West Midlands and Yorkshire.
- Countries like Scotland, England and Denmark use passive registration systems, meaning the relationship between diagnosis of cancer and subsequent death is established through the routine linkage of death certificate data with cancer records.
- France has an active system – linkage with the death certificate requires someone to chase up the appropriate information and death certificates are not public documents in France.
- There is a five-year survival rate difference between countries using active and proactive systems.
- Survival depends on when the patient presents with the illness.
- For many cancers there is a 10%+ variation in five-year survival depending on whether or not the patient comes from an affluent or deprived background.
- Access to linear accelerators has a big influence on survival.

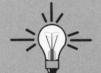

THINK BOX

Given Burn's unpublicised bombshell, why does the cancer clinical community sit back and agree that all this dodgy data adds up to Europe's worst service when it may very well not? Could it be that the gullible government is happy to throw loadsa money into cancer services which is very good for kit, careers and cash in the pocket?

Do we need to treat the information before we treat the system and the patients?

Will we ever know the answer to any of this until public health departments become stand-alone agencies, sharing data and setting real targets for healthcare professionals to work to?

The White Paper, *Our Healthier Nation*, set out a commitment to cut the death rates from cancer in people under 75 by at least a fifth by 2010, aiming, in particular, to improve the health of the worst off. The National Cancer Plan aims to improve cancer services across the whole country.

There will be an extra £570 million a year for cancer services by 2003/04, plus a substantial investment in extra specialist cancer staff. The six medical specialties that contribute most substantially to cancer services, for example, will increase by 24% by 2003/04.

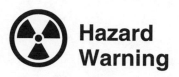 **Hazard Warning**

Perhaps we'd be better off investing in some decent data?

SECTION 12

Coronary heart disease

The burden of coronary heart disease (CHD) is higher and has fallen less in the UK than in many other countries. It kills more than 110 000 people a year in England and death rates are three times higher among manual workers than managers.

CHD is common, frequently fatal and largely preventable.

So get off the couch, stop eating deep pan Hawaiian pizzas, washed down with six beers, pack up the fags, take some exercise and get a grip on your life! End of story!

Not quite but it should be! However, while there's taxpayer's money to be spent . . . well, you know the rest of the story!

Look out for:

- an extra £230 million a year in heart disease services by 2003/04
- an extra £120 million of capital funding from the Treasury Capital Modernisation Fund over the two years to March 2002
- an increase in the number of cardiologists by about 10% each year from 1999/2000, building to a total of 685 by 2003/04, an increase of 47%
- an increase in the number of cardiothoracic surgeons by some 4.5% over the next few years due to the number of trainees currently in the pipeline.

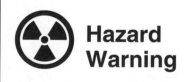 **Hazard Warning**

There's no way this can happen until primary care IT issues are sorted. Doing it by hand with all those horrible Lloyd George folders . . . Ugh!

In future, all patients with established heart disease, or at significant risk of developing it, will receive advice and treatment to reduce their risk of death, heart attack, heart failure and other problems. By 2003, all practices will have disease management registers in place, will be actively managing patients at risk of CHD, and should have clinical audit data demonstrating this.

By 2003, rapid access chest pain clinics will be established right across the country to reassure the pizza eaters, beer drinkers and smokers that within two weeks all patients with new onset chest pain (that their GP thinks might be due to angina) will be assessed!

Now here's a really interesting new development – clot-busting drugs (thrombolysis) should be given within 60 minutes of calling for professional help in the case of a suspected heart attack. This only happens in about one case in 10.

There will be three reforms to improve so-called 'call-to-needle' times.

1 the immediate priority is to improve ambulance response times because every minute counts – arriving one minute early after heart attack gives an extra 11 days of life. By 2001, the ambulance service should achieve first response to 75% of Category A calls within eight minutes. This progress on ambulance response times could save up to 1800 lives a year.

> Increases in traffic and road congestion make this a difficult target to meet. Better fleet management and motorcycles may be part of the answer in some parts of the country. But what if you happen to be in the last 25%?

> How much 'redesign' does it take to organise this? Surely not three years?

2 By 2003, as services are redesigned, 75% of eligible people will receive thrombolysis within 20 minutes of hospital arrival.

3 There will be a three-year programme to train and equip ambulance paramedics to provide thrombolysis safely for appropriate patients.

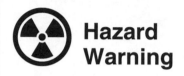

This is the breakthrough!

Waiting lists for cardiac surgery are so long because of chronic NHS under provision in this area. Approx 450 coronary artery bypass grafts per million head of population are carried out in the NHS per annum and approx 375 percutaneous transluminal coronary angioplasty, against a National Service Framework target of at least 750 per million for each procedure per annum.

☢ Hazard Warning

The National Service Framework sets out a series of staged aims to expand capacity for heart services and reduce waits *but* it's wholly dependent on hitting the staffing targets.

SECTION 13

Mental Health Services

For so long the Cinderella service of the NHS. What can we expect?

Most mental health problems are managed in primary care and one in four GP consultations are with patients with mental health problems. So improving these services will have a major impact on primary care and the health and well-being of the population.

- 1000 new graduate primary care mental health workers, trained in brief therapy techniques of proven effectiveness, will be employed to help GPs manage and treat common mental health problems in all age groups, including children.
- 500 more community mental health staff will be employed to work with GPs and primary care teams; NHS Direct and each A&E department to respond to people who need immediate help.
- Staff will be able to call on crisis resolution teams if necessary.
- By 2004, more than 300 000 people will receive extra help from the new primary care mental health workers.
- 500 000 people will benefit from additional mental health staff working in frontline settings.

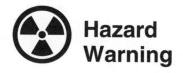 **Hazard Warning**

All very welcome changes and the evidence is 'the faster you respond to a mental health need the greater the chances of minimising the episode'. However, this is a very 'people hungry' policy and success will depend on attracting personnel to that part of the NHS which has always struggled to recruit and retain staff.

When asked, the vast majority of carers focus on the need for mental health services to be provided around the clock, but carers also require time-out to reduce the risk of social isolation which is associated with caring, especially caring for someone with a severe mental illness.

By 2004, 700 more staff will be recruited to increase the breaks available for carers and to strengthen carer support networks. At present, there are very few such staff.

High security hospitals

Some 300–400 patients in high security hospitals do not require that level of security but remain there because no suitable alternative location is available. The government has recently announced an additional £25 million to develop 200 long-term secure beds to allow patients to move on, and to employ 400 additional community staff to provide intensive support when patients are eventually discharged.

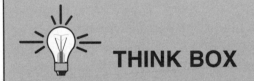

THINK BOX

The average length of stay in a high security hospital such as Broadmoor is surprisingly low – only seven to eight years. If patients are to be given the chance to take up their lives, a large part of the process is recovering social networks and, where possible, family connections. Would a better answer be to close the high security hospitals and build lots of smaller units around the country?

By 2004, up to 400 patients should have moved from the high security hospitals to more appropriate accommodation. Good!

Prison services

At any one time some 5000 people with a serious mental illness will be in prison. It's important to improve the health screening of those received into custody and to identify and provide treatment for prisoners with mental health problems.

Within the new partnerships between the NHS and local prisons, some 300 additional staff will be employed.

- By 2004, 5000 prisoners at any one time should be receiving more comprehensive mental health services in prison.
- All people with severe mental illness will be in receipt of treatment.
- No prisoner with a serious mental illness will leave prison without a care plan and a care co-ordinator.

To ensure that mental health and social care provision can be properly integrated locally, statutory powers will be taken to permit the establishment of combined mental health and social care trusts. Every such trust will be required to establish a Patient Advocate and Liaison Service.

The Mental Health Act (1993) will be reformed to create a new legislative framework reflecting modern patterns of care and treatment for severe mental illness. The present legislation was developed before new approaches to treatment, new drugs and a service aiming to be provided, in the main, in the community.

All very good but what about this . . .

In good nick – isn't there another way?

The benefits of telemedicine for the prison service seem pretty obvious when you think about it. The trouble is, no-one seems to have given it much thought. You can't have folk who are banged up in the nick making visits to the local hospital. Well, that's not quite true because they do – chains, handcuffs, prison guards and the full nine yards. But it upsets the feint-hearted at the clinics and the prisoners don't like the embarrassment of it all either, unless of course they're planning on doing a runner! More importantly, by all accounts, healthcare in prison is not as good as it could be and TMed is one way of improving things – fast.

A recent Home Office Report suggests that prison healthcare should be provided by the NHS. Seems to make sense but some of the problems are not obvious. For example, a prisoner referred to a hospital consultant for care goes on the waiting list like everyone else. But for a variety of reasons prisoners are often shuffled around the prison system, from one prison to another and of course the average frequency of these moves is somewhat shorter than the average NHS waiting list. This means they're moved before they get to the top and in the great snakes and ladders of prison healthcare they slither to the bottom of the waiting list for the nearest hospital to their new 'home'.

Some estimates reckon that about 35% of inmates suffer some form of mental illness. Mental health remains the responsibility of their 'home' mental health Trust, not the host Trust covering the prison area. Not all need specialist care but many do. So, every day, British Rail makes a nice little profit from shuffling consultant psychiatrists, social workers and psychiatric nurses around the country to visit their patients. Nonsense.

With the greatest respect to the Prison Service it's not the best staffed organisation and does seem to like the odd 'away day' disguised as industrial action. Manning levels are very tight and a bout of flu among prison staff can have the same effect. This means prisoners are unexpectedly banged up and many miss hospital appointments as a result. Who knows how often it happens. And even if they do get there, taking a prisoner to a hospital in itself consumes a lot of manpower and resources, meaning that the rest of the prison may be 'locked down'.

As many as one in five prisoners has a serious drug addiction problem. A prison might seem an obvious place to detox. Not so however as detox takes constant monitoring and care – seldom available in prisons at present. By all accounts a steady supply of illegal substances is readily available inside prisons and it's not unknown for a 'straight' prisoner to acquire a habit whilst they are in the nick.

From this summary of the problems the prison service faces you don't have to be Einstein to realise that TMed could, and increasingly will, play a part in improving the healthcare of prisoners.

This is an extract from *The Telemedicine Tool Kit* by Dr John Navein and yours truly, and published by Radcliffe Medical Press. Please buy a copy as John has just moved house and can do with the cash! Thank you.

SECTION 14

The Gold Card members of the NHS

Older people make up the largest single group of patients using the NHS as people over 65 account for two-thirds of hospital patients and 40% of all emergency admissions. Too often they are treated in inappropriate acute hospital settings because there is nowhere else.

Older people also worry about the prospect of deteriorating health, and can be anxious that they may not receive the care they need, sometimes simply because of their age.

They are also distressed when we fail to respect their dignity and privacy, a problem which can occur at home or in a nursing home, as well as on the hospital ward.

> A fit, elderly lady who was in need of the usual maintenance visits ladies of indeterminate 80s make to their GPs, told me that on each of the previous seven occasions she had visited her GP, she had seen a different person.
>
> She was seen by other partners and locums and has the misfortune of being looked after by a bright doctor who is keen on PCGs and has been voted in as the chair. He's always away at meetings.
>
> I suggested she try to get on the list of a less ambitious doctor!

By 2004, the government is making available annually an additional £1.4 billion for new investment in health and social services for older people.

Will this help to:

- assure standards of care?
- extend access to services?

- promote independence in old age?
- ensure fairness in funding?
- . . . and put the elderly, their needs and wishes at the centre of service delivery?

The new National Care Standards Commission has been established to drive up standards across domiciliary and residential care and begins work in 2002.

Later in 2000, the Department of Health will publish a new National Service Framework which will set out clear standards for the services that older people use, including those for stroke, falls and mental health problems.

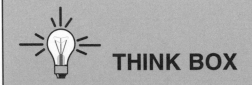

THINK BOX

Stroke victims and mental health service users are often lumped together into 'services for the elderly'. Let's not forget that many stroke victims and mental health sufferers are not elderly and have vastly different needs and perspectives.

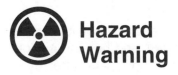

Hazard Warning

Major concerns have been expressed about ageism in the NHS, specifically with respect to resuscitation policies.

All NHS organisations will be required to establish and implement local resuscitation policies based on the guidelines published by the BMA, the Royal College of Nursing and the Resuscitation Council (UK), and to include compliance with these policies in their clinical audit programme.

However, the policy is not universally accepted by doctors and an alternative set of guidelines is available. Set against the background of the human rights legislation that arrived on our doorstep on 2 October 2000, this is a policy that may well have to be looked at again.

Health services in partnership with social services and other agencies will need to recognise the specific needs of older people when caring for them:

- demonstrate proper respect for the autonomy, dignity and privacy of older people
- treat the person, not just the most acute symptoms, by taking account of the full needs of older people, including the importance of good nutrition, maintaining tissue viability and enabling the older person to remain as active as possible while in hospital
- make high-quality palliative and supportive care available to those older people who need it

What about palliative care for younger people?

- ensure good clinical practice that recognises the complexities of caring for older people, e.g. by promoting the good practice recommendations contained in the most recent report of the National Confidential Enquiry into Peri-operative Deaths

Important reading if you are involved in these services

By 2001, the NHS will pilot an NHS retirement health check – a free health check on retirement – to review any current treatment and identify any further potential health problems. And breast screening will be extended to cover all women aged 65 to 70 years as soon as possible.

By April 2002, health and social services will be working much more closely with the introduction of a single assessment process for health and social

Make a Note

Consider a set of joint protocols for older people who are most vulnerable, e.g. those who live alone or those recently bereaved or perhaps those recently discharged from hospital or entering residential or nursing care.

care, with protocols to be agreed locally between health and social services.

Care Direct is a new service to be developed entirely for the benefit of older people. It will provide faster access to care, advice and support – information and advice about health, social care, housing, pensions and benefits by telephone, drop-in centres, on-line and outreach services.

> On-line services for the elderly? A joke? No, a good idea! Many elderly people are now using e-mail systems that come as part of the Sky TV digital package, and for relatives anxious to find out what help they can get from the NHS, the Internet is often the first port of call.

It seems to me that the one thing elderly people really want is to get home and keep their independence. The Plan appears to recognise this and NHS and local social services will support older people to make a faster recovery from illness, encouraging independence rather than institutional care, and providing reliable, high-quality on-going support at home.

The Plan provides an extra £900 million by 2003/04 for investment in intermediate care and related services to promote independence and improved quality of care for older people. This is, along with the additional £150 million made available this year, aimed at:

- promoting independence through active recovery and rehabilitation services with an extra 5000 intermediate care beds and a further 1700 supported intermediate care places – together this could benefit around 150 000 more older people each year

> All this is 'people rich' and a lot will depend on success with recruitment and retention policies.

- preventing unnecessary admission to hospital with extra rapid response teams and other forms of admission prevention benefiting around 70 000 more people each year
- enabling 50 000 more people to live independently at home through additional home care and other support
- 50% more people will benefit from community equipment services ranging from simple care equipment and adaptations (e.g. grab rails and

pressure relief mattresses), to more sophisticated equipment such as fall alarms and remote sensor devices

- extending carers' respite services, benefiting a further 75 000 carers and those they care for.

Here it comes, the nitty-gritty issue

Through these changes and extra investment in intermediate care, older people will be able to maintain their health and independence much more effectively, and remain in their own homes wherever possible.

However, for some people, residential or nursing care is the right option. This brings us to the thorny issue of long-term funding. People who need nursing care in nursing homes may have to pay for it, whereas it's free in every other setting. Many people fear having to sell their own homes to pay for their care.

In 1997, the government established a Royal Commission on Long-Term Care to specifically examine these issues and to make proposals for reform.

Many of the Commission's recommendations, such as the establishment of a National Care Standards Commission, have already been actioned. A full response to the Royal Commission is being published separately and is a 'must read' if you are involved in these services. However, to save you time . . .

The government intends to action the following proposals:

- From April 2001: for the first three months from admission to residential and nursing home care, the value of a person's home will be disregarded from the means testing rules. This is intended to give people a breathing space in which to consider their position and allow the possibility of a return home.

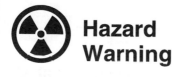 **Hazard Warning**

Sadly, the majority of elderly people who enter nursing home care do not return home. So as welcome as the respite is, it's not a lot of help – although, in fairness, this is thought to benefit around 30 000 people each year.

- The capital limits used when assessing someone's ability to contribute to the costs of their care will be restored to the 1996 value and will be kept under review.

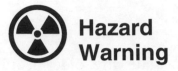 **Hazard Warning**

Many argue that the capital limits in 1996 were insufficiently generous then and do little to improve the situation now.

- Statutory guidance is to be issued to councils to reduce the current unacceptable variations in charges for home care. This could benefit many of the 500 000 people who receive home care each year.

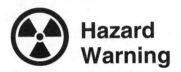 **Hazard Warning**

Many of the charges are set by local authority members trying to balance their council's budget. Arriving at a uniformity of charging may be much more difficult in practice than it looks in theory.

- From October 2001: subject to a decision by Parliament, nursing care provided in nursing homes will be fully funded by the NHS.

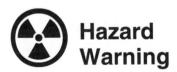 **Hazard Warning**

This is the big one and the decision that split the members of the Royal Commission, causing a row. The Commission recommended that all care should be paid for and here's what they said in the report.

This doesn't excuse you from reading the whole thing – it's important that you do!

'The cost of care for those individuals who need it should be split between living costs, housing costs and personal care. Personal care should be available after an assessment, according to need and paid for from general taxation – the rest should be subject to a co-payment according to needs.'

And here's the first part of the government's response:

'The government believes this would not be the most effective targeting of resources. At present, personal care is provided on a means tested basis through local councils. Making personal care free for everyone carries a substantial cost and one that is difficult to predict for the future. It would demand substantial resources without necessarily improving services.'

In other words: no – it'll cost too much! Here's the conundrum. When is a personal service a health service and when is a health service a personal service?

Take the case of an elderly man in a residential nursing home suffering from Alzheimer's disease. He's unaware of his surroundings, confused, incontinent and unable to concentrate long enough to feed himself.

He's in general good health and requires no medication other than a sedative at bedtime.

However, he needs constant attention as he's likely to wander and harm himself. He's unable to bathe or dress himself and needs help with incontinence aids. Without help feeding, he will starve.

None of these vital needs comes into the category of nursing care – they are all personal services and these services are means tested . . . you can see the problem.

- From April 2002: payment of the Residential Allowance will cease for new care home residents and the resources will be transferred to local authorities.

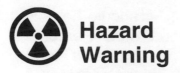

Hazard Warning

At present these resources can encourage councils to place older people in residential care and to select independent sector homes. The individual does not benefit from the money as the local authority usually recoups it. In future this money will be available to promote independence and active rehabilitation for older people.

Those who entered residential care before April 1993 can expect extra help and financial support as local councils become responsible for their assessment, care management and financial support. This change will benefit around 65 000 people and will ensure that people cannot be moved against their will unless there are compelling reasons to do so.

Look out for an important change in the regulations that will allow councils to help older people who entered care before the 1993 community care changes and who face eviction from their care home because they cannot pay the fees. A new grant to local authorities to expand loan schemes should help to ensure that no old person will be forced to sell their home against their will when they go into long-term care. This new system promises to be fairer and clearer.

SECTION 15

What do you think of the show so far?

Something for everyone? A patchwork? A collection of aspirations? A plan? What do you think and how do you rate it?

Is this how you would like to see the future of the NHS?

Yup!

- Clinical priorities over political priorities and all patients with serious problems treated within three months in the NHS or have it paid for in the private sector?
- Access to information about waiting times, treatments and success rates of hospitals?
- Dedicated surgical units for treatments such as cataracts and hip replacements, with some procedures performed by GPs?
- Special funds and a committee dedicated to working on the advice of NICE to end postcode variations in treatment?
- An independent review body for NHS appointments?
- More specialisation among GPs and less micro-management of the NHS?
- Tax incentives to encourage greater use of the private sector?

If you ticked 'yes' to these, you'll love Tory policy on health! The points are taken from William Hague's speech to the Centre for Policy Studies, the day before the PM introduced the NHS Plan to Parliament.

I just included it in the interest of balance. Wicked, I know. Sorry!

SECTION 16

Reform watch: at a glance

The problem with a package as big as the NHS Plan is that it's easy to overlook the targets as the aims and ambitions get lost in the effort of the working day. Every once in a while take a step back and think about your role in helping to hit the targets – do you think they are attainable and just as important? See if the targets have been hit.

You have a role
Done
Not done
Never will be!

For the NHS
- Reduce the maximum wait for an outpatient appointment to three months and the maximum wait for inpatient treatment to six months by the end of 2005.
- Patients will receive treatment at a time that suits them in accordance with their clinical need: two-thirds of all outpatient appointments and inpatient elective admissions will be pre-booked by 2003/04, with 100% pre-booking by 2005.
- Guaranteed access to a primary care professional within 24 hours and to a primary care doctor within 48 hours by 2004.
- To secure year-on-year improvements in patient satisfaction including standards of cleanliness and food, as measured by independently audited surveys.

You have a role
Done
Not done
Never will be!

- Reduce substantially the mortality rates from major killers by 2010:
  - from heart disease by at least 40% in people under 75
  - from cancer by at least 20% in people under 75
  - and from suicide and undetermined injury by at least 20%.
- Key to the delivery of this target will be implementing the NSFs for CHD and mental health and the National Cancer Plan – the objective is to narrow the health gap in childhood and throughout life between socio-economic groups and between the most deprived areas and the rest of the country. Specific national targets will be developed with stakeholders and experts early in 2001.
- The cost of care commissioned from Trusts which perform well against indicators of fair access, quality and responsiveness, will become the benchmark for the NHS. Everyone will be expected to reach the level of the best over the next five years, with agreed milestones for 2003/04.

For the NHS in partnership with social services
- Provide high-quality pre-admission and rehabilitation care to older people to help them live as independently as possible by reducing preventable hospitalisation and ensuring year-on-year reductions in delays in moving people over 75 on from hospital.
- Monitor progress in the Performance Assessment Framework and increase the participation of problem drug users in drug treatment programmes by 55% by 2004, and 100% by 2008.

You have a role
Done
Not done
Never will be!

For social services
Improve the life chances for children in care.
- Improving the level of education, training and employment outcomes for care leavers aged 19, so that levels for this group are at least 75% of those achieved by all young people in the same area by March 2004.
- Increasing the percentage of children in care who achieve at least five grade A to C GCSEs to 15% by 2004.
- Giving them the care and guidance needed to narrow the gap by 2004 between the proportion of children in care and their peers who are cautioned or convicted.
- Maximising the contribution adoption can make in providing permanent families for children – a specific target will be set for adoption services.

The next steps
Implementation of this NHS Plan begins immediately.
- During August 2000, new resources to increase the number of heart operations will be allocated to the NHS.
- By September 2000, the Modernisation Board will be in place.
- By autumn 2000, the new NHS Chief Executive will be appointed.
- In the autumn, the Modernisation Board will agree and publish a detailed implementation programme for the NHS Plan.
- In the autumn, health authorities will be provided with three-year allocations.

SECTION 17

All the targets:
the complete list

Here's a timeline of the benchmarks and targets in the plan. Check off the ones that affect you and cross 'em off when you've done it.

Cut out these pages and pin them on your notice board to show how smart you are!

 Make a Note

Think about how you'll be cascading the targets and implementation strategies to colleagues and staff – what's the plan?

This impacts on me/where I work/what I do
Phew, Done it!

Implementation of this NHS Plan begins immediately

- By September 2000, the Modernisation Board will be in place.
- By autumn 2000, the new NHS Chief Executive will be appointed.
- During August 2000, new resources to increase the number of heart operations will be allocated to the NHS.
- National standards for cleanliness will form part of the NHS Performance Assessment Framework. Every hospital's performance will be measured against these standards by the end of 2000.
- The National Cancer Plan to be published in autumn 2000.
- A NSF for older people's services will be published in autumn 2000.
- By the end of 2000 NHS Direct will have gone nationwide.
- The number of cardiologists will increase by some 10% each year from 1999/2000.
- Nine new hospital schemes will be given the go-ahead in 2001, worth £1.3 billion.

By 2001

- A 24-hour NHS catering service with a new NHS menu, designed by leading chefs. It will cover continental breakfast, cold drinks and snacks at mid-morning; in the afternoon, light lunchtime meals; and an improved two-course evening dinner. This will be a minimum standard for all hospitals.
- A national franchise for NHS catering will be examined to ensure hospital food is provided by organisations with a national reputation for high quality and customer satisfaction.
- Half of all hospitals will have new 'ward housekeepers' in place by 2004 to ensure that the quality, presentation and quantity of meals meet patient needs; that patients, particularly elderly people, are able to eat the meals on offer; and that the service patients receive is genuinely available

round-the-clock. Dieticians will advise and check on nutritional values in hospital food. Patients' views will be measured as part of the Performance Assessment Framework and there will be unannounced inspections of the quality of hospital food. An extra £10m a year will be made available to deliver these improvements.

- The new model of nurse education and training as described in the nursing, midwifery and health visiting strategy, *Making a Difference*, with its emphasis on improving access, developing practical skills earlier in training and with stepping off points at the end of the first year, will be rolled out nationwide. By autumn 2001, 85% of all nurse training organisations will be operating the new arrangements.

- From April 2001, the government will introduce a National Health Performance Fund building up to £500m a year by 2003/04. The fund, which will be held and distributed regionally, will allow incentives worth on average £5m for each HA area to be available to reward progress against annually agreed objectives.

- By the end of 2005, waiting lists for hospital appointments and admission will be abolished and replaced with booking systems giving all patients a choice of a convenient time, within a guaranteed maximum waiting time. As a first step towards this all hospitals will, by April 2001, have booking systems in place covering two procedures within their major specialties.

By 2002

- All GP practices will be connected to NHSnet.
- 1000 of the 1100 extra medical school places that have already been announced are expected to come on-stream.

This impacts on me/where I work/what I do
Phew, Done it!

- In social services, £50m a year will be available from April 2002 to reward improved social services joint working arrangements based on measuring performance from 2001.
- Nearly a third of all GPs to be working to PMS contracts.
- From 2002, the government will centrally fund all specialist registrar posts, provided that agreement can be reached with the medical Royal Colleges and other bodies on curricula and criteria for training recognition.
- The new model of nurse education and training, described in *Making a Difference*, with its emphasis on improving access, developing practical skills earlier in training and with stepping off points at the end of the first year, will be rolled out nationwide.
- By autumn 2001, 85% of all nurse training organisations will be operating the new arrangements. By autumn 2002, it will be standard across the whole of England.
- Pain clinics will be established right across the country to assess, within two weeks, all patients with new onset chest pain, which their GP thinks might be due to angina. There will be 50 such clinics by April 2001, 100 by April 2002.
- It will be a pre-condition of qualification to deliver patient care in the NHS that an individual has demonstrated competence in communication with patients.
- By April 2002, every hospital will have senior sisters and charge nurses who are easily identifiable to patients and who will be accountable for a group of wards (Matron).
- The GMC's mandatory five-yearly revalidation process is likely to begin in 2002 – if it survives?
- An NHS-wide Patient Advocacy and Liaison Service (PALS) will be established in every Trust, beginning with every major hospital. The national annual budget will be around £10m.

This impacts on me/where I work/what I do
Phew, Done it!

- From 2002, when a patient's operation is cancelled by the hospital on the day of surgery for non-clinical reasons, the hospital will have to offer another binding date within a maximum of the next 28 days, or fund the patient's treatment at the time and hospital of the patient's choice.
- All NHS Direct sites will refer people, where appropriate, to help from their local pharmacy and there will be better out-of-hours pharmacy services.
- To underpin national work on cutting inequalities by 2002, development of a new health poverty index that combines data about health status, access to health services, uptake of preventive services and the opportunities to pursue and maintain good health, e.g. access to affordable nutritious food, physical activity and a safe, clean environment.
- There will be new single, integrated public health groups across NHS Regional Offices and government offices of the regions. Accountable through the Regional Director of Public Health to both the Director of the government office for the region and the NHS Regional Director, they will enable regeneration of regions to embrace health as well as environment, transport and inward investment.
- There will be a Healthy Communities Collaborative to spread best practice under the aegis of the new Modernisation Agency, using evidence from the Health Development Agency and the successful formula already in place in the Cancer Collaborative and the Primary Care Collaborative.
- NICE will issue guidance by 2002 on how best to organise urological, haematological and head and neck cancer services and supportive/palliative care. It will also update existing guidance for breast, bowel and lung cancer services. Implementation will be rolled out as the guidance becomes available.

This impacts on me/where I work/what I do

Phew, Done it!

- An extra £120m of capital funding from the Treasury Capital Modernisation Fund over the two years to March 2002, to expand capacity and modernise services.
- The new National Care Standards Commission starts its work in 2002 to drive up standards across domiciliary and residential care.
- Local services will streamline their local assessment processes, recognising the complexity of what some older people require. By April 2002, a single assessment process for health and social care, with protocols to be agreed locally between health and social services.
- During 2002, older people and, where appropriate, their carers will be involved in agreeing a personal care plan, which they will hold.
- From April 2002, payment of the Residential Allowance will cease for new care home residents and the resources will be transferred to local authorities.

By 2003

- 38 major developments. Over half of these will be open to the public by 2003/04 and the remainder will be under construction.
- An extra £250m will be invested in information technology in 2003/04.
- By April 2003, all NHS employers are expected to be accredited as putting the Improving Working Lives standard into practice.
- More help with personal development and training – an extra £140m by 2003/04 to ensure that all professional staff are supported in keeping their skills up to date and to provide access to learning for all NHS staff without a professional qualification.
- Extend occupational health services, already a requirement in hospitals, with

This impacts on me/where I work/what I do
Phew, Done it!

£6m in 2001/02, building to £8m in 2003/04 for community Trusts, GPs and their staff. Standards for occupational health services for NHS staff will be included in the Improving Working Lives standard.

- Intermediate care and related services – £900m investment by 2003/04 to promote independence and improve the quality of care for older people.
- Local authorities, health authorities, PCGs and PCTs will receive incentive payments to encourage and reward joint working. In the case of health organisations it will be through the National Performance Fund.
- In social services £50m a year will be available from April 2002 to reward improved social services joint working arrangements based on measuring performance from 2001. From April 2003, the fund will rise to £100m.
- To help people take on these new roles there will be an extra £140m by 2003/04 to support a major programme of training and development for all staff.
- Following the review of the existing weighted capitation formula used to distribute NHS funding, reducing inequalities will be a key criterion for allocating NHS resources to different parts of the country.
- A free and nationally available translation and interpretation service will be available from all NHS premises through NHS Direct.
- There will be a leadership programme for health visitors and community nurses to be run by the new NHS Leadership Centre.
- Cancer services – an extra £570m a year by 2003/04.
- The six medical specialties that contribute most substantially to cancer services, for example, will increase by 24% by 2003/04.

This impacts on me/where I work/what I do

Phew, Done it!

- A Cancer Services Collaborative is working with nine cancer networks across the country to streamline all stages in the pathway of care. The new Modernisation Agency will extend this approach to all cancer networks by 2003.
- Heart disease services – an extra £230m a year by 2003/04.
- The number of cardiologists will increase by some 10% each year from 1999/2000, building to a total of some 685 by 2003/04 – an increase of 47%.
- The number of trainees currently in the pipeline means that cardiothoracic surgeons will increase by some 4.5% each year for the next few years – an increase of 19% by 2003/04.
- All practices will have disease management registers in place, be actively managing patients at risk of CHD, and have clinical audit data demonstrating this.
- Rapid access chest pain clinics will be established right across the country to assess, within two weeks, all patients with new onset chest pain, which their GP thinks might be due to angina. There will be 50 such clinics by April 2001, 100 by April 2002, with national rollout being completed in 2003.
- 75% of eligible people will receive thrombolysis within 20 minutes of hospital arrival as services are redesigned.
- An extra annual investment of over £300m by 2003/04 to fast-forward the National Service Framework.
- All 20 000 people estimated to need assertive outreach will be receiving these services.
- Intermediate care and related services – an extra £900m by 2003/04 to promote independence and improved quality of care for older people.
- Two-thirds of all outpatient appointments and inpatient elective admissions will be pre-booked by 2003/04. Patients will receive treatment at a time that suits them in accordance with their clinical need.

This impacts on me/where I work/what I do
Phew, Done it!

By 2004

- 7000 extra NHS beds.
- 20 Diagnostic and Treatment Centres developed. Eight will be fully operational treating approx 200 000 patients a year.
- The NHS will have cleared at least a quarter of its £3.1bn maintenance backlog.
- Up to 3000 family doctors' premises will be substantially refurbished or replaced.
- 500 one-stop primary care centres.
- Equipment to improve cancer, renal and heart disease services, a +£300m investment.
- Half of all hospitals will have new 'ward housekeepers' in place to ensure that the quality, presentation and quantity of meals meets patient needs; that patients, particularly elderly people, are able to eat the meals on offer; and that the service patients receive is genuinely available round-the-clock.
- Bedside televisions and telephones will be available in every major hospital.
- Access to electronic personal medical records for patients.
- Electronic prescribing of medicines and easier access to repeat prescriptions.
- 7500 more consultants.
- 2000 more general practitioners.
- 20 000 more nurses.
- Over 6500 more therapists and other health professionals.
- Expect more than 45 000 new nurses and midwives to come out of training.
- Over 13 000 therapists and other health professionals.
- 5500 more nurses, midwives and health visitors being trained each year.
- 4450 more therapists and other key professional staff being trained.
- 1000 more specialist registrars – the key feeder grade for consultants – targeting key specialties.

This impacts on me/where I work/what I do

Phew, Done it!

- 450 more doctors training for general practice.
- NHS-sponsored on-site nursery provision funding, building up to an additional investment of over £30m.
- There will be provision for on-site nurseries at around 100 hospitals provided at an average subsidy of £30 per place per week.
- Expect all PCGs to have become PCTs.
- There will be 2000 more GPs and 450 more GPs in training.
- 3000 family doctors' premises including 500 new primary care centres – a £1bn investment programme.
- The revised national contract for GPs should reflect the emphasis on quality and improved outcomes inherent in the PMS approach. Both local PMS and national arrangements are set to operate within a single contractual framework.
- A new national PMS contract will be introduced into which all single-handed practices will be transferred by 2004.
- Consultants working in the NHS will have:
  - a major investment in equipment, IT and facilities
  - a 30% expansion in consultant numbers with further increases in the pipeline
  - expansion in medical school places and specialist registrar posts.
- An increase in the number of consultants in receipt of a superannuable bonus from under one half of all consultants at present to around two-thirds, and to double the proportion of consultants who receive annual bonuses of £5000 or more.
- The majority of NHS staff will be working under agreed protocols identifying how common conditions should be handled and which staff can best handle them.
- A majority of nurses should be able to prescribe.
- There will be around 1000 nurse consultants.

This impacts on me/where I work/what I do
Phew, Done it!

- Provision of health information via digital TV as well as via the telephone and Internet. By then there will be over 500 NHS Direct information points providing touchscreen information and advice about health and the health service, in places like shopping centres and railway stations.
- A single phone call to NHS Direct will be a one-stop gateway to out-of-hours healthcare, passing on calls, where necessary, to the appropriate GP co-operative or deputising service.
- Every PCG or PCT will have schemes in place so that people get more help from pharmacists in using their medicines.
- Patients will be able to see a primary care professional within 24 hours and a GP within 48 hours.
- Patients who currently have to go to hospital will be able to have tests and treatment in primary care centres as staff numbers and skills expand.
- Consultants who previously worked only in hospitals will be delivering approx four million outpatient consultations in primary care and community settings.
- Up to 1000 specialist GPs will be taking referrals from fellow GPs for conditions in specialties such as ophthalmology, orthopaedics, dermatology and ear, nose and throat surgery. They will also be able to undertake diagnostic procedures such as endoscopy.
- An end to widespread bed blocking.
- No-one should be waiting more than four hours in A&E from arrival to admission, transfer or discharge.
- To improve further the equitable distribution of GPs and primary care staff, there will be 200 new PMS schemes created principally in disadvantaged communities by 2004.
- There will be an expansion of Sure Start projects to cover a third of children aged under four years living in poverty. Spending will rise to around £500m.

This impacts on me/where I work/what I do

Phew, Done it!

- A new National School Fruit Scheme where every child in nursery and aged four to six in infant schools will be entitled to a free piece of fruit each school day, as part of a national campaign to improve the diet of children.
- (Pilot) A five-a-day programme to increase fruit and vegetable consumption.
- (Pilot) Work with industry, including producers as well as retailers, to increase provision and access to fruit and vegetables. Local initiatives, where necessary, to establish local food co-operatives.
- (Pilot) Initiatives with the food industry, including manufacturers and caterers, to improve the overall balance of diet including salt, fat and sugar in food. Working with the Food Standards Agency.
- (Pilot) Local action to tackle obesity and physical inactivity, informed by advice from the new Health Development Agency on what works.
- (Pilot) A hospital nutrition policy to improve the outcome of care for patients, aiming to reduce dependency on intravenous feeding regimes.
- (Pilot) An alcohol misuse strategy.
- A new NHS Cancer Research Network will be fully implemented by 2004.
- More than 300 000 people will receive extra help from the new primary care mental health workers and around 500 000 people will benefit from additional mental health staff working in frontline settings.
- All young people who experience a first episode of psychosis, such as schizophrenia, will receive the early and intensive support they need.
- All people in contact with specialist mental health services will be able to access crisis resolution services at any time.
- Services will be redesigned to ensure there are women-only day centres in every health authority.

This impacts on me/where I work/what I do
Phew, Done it!

- 700 more staff will be recruited to increase the breaks available for carers, and to strengthen carer support networks.
- Up to 400 patients should have moved from the high security hospitals to more appropriate accommodation.
- 5000 prisoners at any one time should be receiving more comprehensive mental health services in prison.
- An additional 140 new secure places and 75 specialist rehabilitation hostel places will be provided for people with severe personality disorder, employing almost 400 extra staff.
- A further £360m will be invested to help people meet the costs of their residential and nursing home care.
- Guaranteed access to a primary care professional within 24 hours and to a primary care doctor within 48 hours.
- Increase the participation of problem drug users in drug treatment programmes by 55%.
- Improving the level of education, training and employment outcomes for care leavers aged 19, so that levels for this group are at least 75% of those achieved by all young people in the same area by March 2004.
- To narrow the gap between the proportion of children in care and their peers who are cautioned or convicted.
- Improving the educational attainment of children and young people in care by increasing, from 6% in 1998 to 15% in 2004, the proportion of children leaving care aged 16 and over with five GCSEs at grades A to C.

By 2005
- Electronic booking of appointments for patient treatment.
- Have facilities for telemedicine allowing patients to electronically connect with staff for advice.

This impacts on me/where I work/what I do
Phew, Done it!

- Every patient will be able to book a hospital appointment and elective admission will give them a choice of convenient date and time rather than being assigned a time by the hospital.
- Three months maximum wait for outpatients.
- Six months maximum wait for an operation, falling to three months thereafter.
- By the end of 2005, waiting lists for hospital appointments and admission will be abolished and replaced with booking systems giving all patients a choice of convenient time, within a guaranteed maximum waiting time.
- As a first step towards this all hospitals will by April 2001 have booking systems in place covering two procedures within their major specialties.
- Assuming GP referrals remain broadly in line with the current trend in the growth of referrals, then the maximum waiting time for a routine outpatient appointment will be halved from over six months now to three months. Urgent cases will continue to be treated much faster in accordance with clinical need. As a result, expect the average waiting time for an outpatient appointment to fall to five weeks.
- The maximum wait for inpatient treatment will be cut from 18 months now to six months. Urgent cases will continue to be treated much faster in accordance with clinical need. As a result, expect the average waiting time for inpatient treatment to fall from three months to seven weeks.
- Commitment to reducing the proportion of people under the age of 25 reporting the use of class A drugs by 25%.
- Increase the number of problem drug misusers in treatment by 66%.
- Authoritative guidance will be available from NICE on new standards for all aspects of NHS cancer care, with implementation taking place in line with the expansion in the workforce.

This impacts on me/where I work/what I do

Phew, Done it!

- Reduce the maximum wait for an outpatient appointment to three months and the maximum wait for inpatient treatment to six months by the end of 2005.
- The eventual objective is to reduce the maximum wait for any stage of treatment to three months.
- Two-thirds of all outpatient appointments and inpatient elective admissions will be pre-booked by 2003/04, with 100% pre-booking by 2005.

And by 2010!

- The redesigned NHS to be patient centred, offering a personalised service. (*It's already happening in some places and by 2010 it will be commonplace.*)
- Over 100 new hospitals.
- £7bn of new capital investment through an extended role for PFI.
- Full implementation of the government's teenage pregnancy strategy, bringing about a 15% reduction in the rate of teenage conception – this is consistent with the longer-term target of reducing the rate of teenage conception by half by 2010.
- Approx 55 000 fewer women will be smoking in pregnancy.
- At least 1.5m smokers will have given up smoking.
- Cut the death rate from cancer in people under 75 by at least a fifth, aiming, in particular, to improve the health of the worst off.
- Five-year cancer survival rates will compare with the best in Europe.
- Reduce substantially the mortality rates from major killers – from heart disease by at least 40% in people under 75; from cancer by at least 20% in people under 75; and from suicide and undetermined injury by at least 20%.